BLOOD SUGAR IN CHECK

7 Steps to Health and Happiness with Diabetes

Rockant, Inc.

Rockville, Maryland, USA

Published March 2019

ISBN-13: 978-0-578-47118-1

Disclaimer

Moral Support: Ann Lawless

Book Coach: Dr. Angela Lauria

Cover Design: Flor Figueroa

Photography: Eugene Lawless

Developmental Editor: Ora North

Managing Editor: Bethany Davis

Manuscript Cleanup: Erica L. James

Proofreading: Jennifer Hoffner

Dedication

For Monika

This is the book I wish we'd had when we were diagnosed.

Andrew Lawless

Contents

Foreword by Daniele Hargenrader

As I read through *Blood Sugar in Check*, I couldn't help but feel a familiar sense of kindred connection to Andrew and all of my brothers and sisters out there performing the lifelong forced dance with diabetes. Although everyone has their own unique experiences living with diabetes, we all share a common bond of understanding the hard work required to keep ourselves alive, of empathy for and acceptance of our fellow humans who live with this disease.

I'm currently in my 28th year living with type 1. Creating a conscious, intentional, and sustainable way to live happy and healthy with diabetes is, and has always been, 20% medical and 80% mental for me. This is also true for the thousands of people I've been blessed to work with over the past 8 years who have all types of diabetes. But the sad and scary thing is that medical doctors generally do not address the mental, emotional, and spiritual (in the medical world a.k.a. psychosocial) aspects of living with a disease that requires 24-7 attention.

Generally speaking, absolutely zero mindset and emotional management tools are given in the doctor's office. All too often we are left feeling overwhelmed and alone, even though the plethora of resources for intelligently managing this crucial aspect of our diabetes care continues to grow every day. Luckily, you are reading one of those resources right now.

Having spent more than 8 years of my type 1 life clinically depressed, on antidepressants, obese, and with an eating disorder, I found my own route out of that personal hell in a time when the Internet was just coming into existence. It eventually became my life's work and led me to finding the path toward fulfilling my dharma, our true purpose for existing in this current time and space. At first, I did this work for myself, and it has evolved to serving others. I will always be grateful for the incredibly valuable lessons I learned and continue to learn when pain is my teacher.

If you are willing to step up and give yourself the gift of mindful self-love through choosing to live in the present, the steps Andrew has laid out for you in this book will undoubtedly lead to feeling more joy and less pain in your relationship with diabetes.

Throughout this book, Andrew prompts you to explore what I agree is the most important factor in changing your relationship with diabetes from one of pain and hopelessness to one of joy and empowerment: your mindset. Your mindset encompasses many things, such as what you believe to be true. It includes the meanings you assign to each and every thing you ever experience, the language you use when talking about yourself and your relationship with your diabetes, and your willingness to explore the life-changing power of choosing to change your mindset if it is no longer serving your overall wellness.

You will recognize each and every area Andrew encourages you to change, because these forces live within us all: self-sabotage, low self-worth, self-doubt, self-deception, and feeling like a burden to those we love. All of these things create a mindset of paralysis, helplessness, hopelessness, and self-pity, which can bring on appalling behavior that creates the quality of our everyday reality of life with diabetes. I speak from years of personal experience.

I may not agree with everything Andrew says, because we all have our own diabetes management practices that work for us individually, but he clearly states that he isn't trying to lead you to blindly adopting his practices. Instead, he guides you through a system that will allow you to create your own sustainable diabetes management system that is all your own, feels empowering, and is a necessary journey to embark on to truly feel confident and capable of being your own best diabetes expert.

This self-exploration is life altering in the best ways possible. There is no doctor or expert or human who can tell you what works best for you; only you can know what works best for you by consciously and intentionally experimenting, exploring, listening to the feedback your mind, body, and spirit are always sending, and course correcting. Through this process your own system emerges. These are all practices of self-love, and they are indeed the only way out of a hellish relationship with your diabetes.

In my teachings and way of life, the terms "self-love" and "mindfulness" are synonymous. You cannot practice self-love without practicing mindfulness, and vice versa. The amount of health and happiness we feel day to day is directly proportional to the amount of self-love we are willing to practice and bestow on ourselves. These practices cultivate and strengthen self-worth, which leads directly to better diabetes management in all areas.

Andrew states, "The space between where you are today and where you want to be is called the gap. Keep on bridging the gap, and you will make changes in all focus areas of your life." Those are wise words. Small, intentional, consistent steps lead to sustainable, joyful habits. Blood Sugar in Check guides you through many small steps that will lead to the lasting changes you are after if you are willing to practice, celebrate your wins no matter how big or small, and learn from your setbacks along the way.

Daniele Hargenrader

Founder of *Diabetes Dominator Coaching*[1] and *The Diabetes Empowerment Summit*[2]
Author of *Unleash Your Inner Diabetes Dominator*
Coauthor of *Love, Forgive, Never Give Up!*

---

[1] Diabetes Dominator Coaching *diabetesdominator.com*
2 The Diabetes Empowerment Summit *diabetesempowermentsummit.com*

Foreword by Dr. Udo Erasmus

When people want to take responsibility for their own health and do natural treatments, there are always three things that I recommend: First, improve nutrient intake. Second, get toxic molecules out of the diet. Third, make sure that digestion works.

Why? Degenerative conditions such as cancer, cardiovascular disease, type II diabetes, and other inflammatory conditions have two causes: Something that should be present (fresh, whole, raw, organic foods; essential nutrients; probiotics; digestive enzymes; fiber) in our food is missing, or something is present that shouldn't be there (poisons, pesticides, pharmaceutical drugs, industrial chemicals, pathogenic microbes, synthetic additives and preservatives, food molecules damaged by processing or destructive food preparation, such as frying). When you deal with those issues, you improve your overall health, well-being, and energy levels.

You can reverse most cases of insulin-resistant, type-II diabetes, provided no permanent damage has been done to vital tissues, by doing the following:

- Ensure optimal intake of all essential nutrients (18 minerals, 13 vitamins, 9 essential amino acids, 2 essential fatty acids), especially emphasizing zinc, chromium, magnesium, and essential fats.

- Reduce the consumption of sugars and sweets; starchy

foods such as grains, bread, and potatoes; processed foods; fruits; and hard (saturated) fats.

- Increase your intake of whole foods and green foods, probiotics, digestive enzymes, and prebiotic fiber.

- Optimize intake of good proteins and good fats, because these supply essential building blocks for body construction that the body cannot make.

- Be active to build muscle, which burn more carbohydrates than fat tissue does.

People with diabetes need a "fuel shift." They do better when they get their energy from essential fats rather than refined carbs, which lead to insulin resistance and leptin resistance, which is believed to be the leading driver of fat gain in humans. Leptin tells the brain that you have enough fat stored and don't need to eat. When you have leptin resistance, your brain erroneously thinks that the body is starving and even changes your physiology and behavior to regain the fat.

The cause of diabetes is temporarily or permanently unhinged carbohydrate metabolism. This is true for both type II and type I diabetes. However, while type II can be reversed by food and lifestyle changes, type I cannot yet be reversed, because we have not learned how to regenerate the insulin-making cells in our pancreas, which have been destroyed by an autoimmune attack. This means that to be effectively managed, type II and type I diabetes require different procedures. These are known to be quite reliable when properly followed.

While the physical procedures for treating both types of diabetes have been laid out by extensive research and documented application, the medical profession has done a poor job of dealing with the equally important mental and emotional aspects of diabetes management.

What makes Andrew's approach unique and important is that he addresses these from his own experiences. He shares what the "gift" of diabetes has made possible for him. He is not only a competent technician, but also the voice of experience here, sharing what he's learned firsthand over 40 years of living a life of excellence with type I diabetes.

Without a forward-looking, life-affirming, positive, inspiring mindset, people with diabetes—like every other human being with any other condition "that flesh is heir to"—will not do what is necessary to thrive in their life rather than merely survive. Let Andrew's ability to turn a problem into a gift rub off on you.

Andrew's approach to training your mind to enjoy your life and keep your blood sugar in check is spot-on. Certain beliefs and behavioral patterns you have acquired over the years can sabotage you when you set out to make a change to a healthier lifestyle. They are hard, but possible, to get out of the system. Letting Andrew coach you will make managing your diabetes more manageable. It helps to have a friend who's been there.

Think about it. Supporting your health means that frying is out, refined oils are out, margarines are out, sugar is out, convenience junk foods are out, and hard fats are out. Foods as nature made them are in. The only oils you should eat are those made with health in mind, rich in both omega-3 and -6 essential fatty acids in the right ratio, minimally processed, and with their minor ingredients still intact. Essential fatty acids lower blood pressure, lower other leading risk factors for cardiovascular disease, and are required for insulin function. They also ensure cell membrane integrity, oxygen metabolism, stamina, and energy levels. That is, by the way, part of the healing standard for all degenerative diseases, including inflammation, cardiovascular disease, arthritis, multiple sclerosis, cancer, and diabetes. It is also the standard for those who are healthy and want to remain healthy.

The health benefits of good oils are clear. But if bacon and bread are current staples of your diet, this is not an easy shift to make. Andrew knows this. Instead of just giving you the usual instructions of counting carbs and determining the dosage of your medication, he focuses from the beginning on building a mindset for a happy and healthy life with diabetes. Only 20% of managing your disease is technical. Another 20% is about the energy that you're able to put into your health management. A whopping 60% of success is your focus, beliefs, and motivation. Once you have that, it's much easier to follow through on the technical advice. With the right attitude, you're good to go.

Andrew knows that most people are still following the recommendations made by government "health experts" in 1979 to eat less fat and more carbohydrates. That wrongheaded advice led to an increase in overweight of the population in 20 years, from 25% to 60%. Obesity more than doubled, childhood obesity more than tripled, and diabetes almost doubled. *Blood Sugar in Check* gives you updated, correct advice that works.

It is easy to say that people are not willing to make changes in their diet to improve health or are not paying attention, but it is more accurate to point out that bad advice keeps people with diabetes who are doing the work from getting the results they seek. So, they quit. In *Blood Sugar in Check*, Andrew focuses on updated, more practical nutritional knowledge. He also points to the missing valid and robust fact that self-doubt and being overwhelmed from managing the disease can be depressing and discouraging. "We can become animals" in survival mode, he writes, rather than thrive.

Andrew shows you what to do, step-by-step. It's reassuring. He also explains why, which helps you understand, develop, and stick to helpful long-term habits. Throughout the book, he writes with compassion borne of his own successes with responsible self-care. His power and confidence come not only from theory, but also from his own experience about how to make significant life-enhancing and life-supporting changes. His compassion especially shows in the discussion about focusing on shifting negative beliefs about diabetes that hold you back and interfere with health and happiness into the belief that your diabetes is a gift and can catapult your quality of life to new heights.

Changing your beliefs helps change your habits. Changing your habits helps you change your health and manage your diabetes. You are not a diabetic. You are life in human form. Remembering what a gift life is puts you in charge and evaporates the temptation to see yourself as a victim of diabetes. Independent of its present state, every body is a terminal condition. That's true for every one of us. Yet within that terminal condition, you are awesome and magnificent. Thinking in line with the lit-up nature of your life makes you sound and gives you the deepest, most meaningful personal feeling.

Eating in line with nature—fresh, whole, raw, organic, not too much, mostly plants plus a B12 supplement—best supports the health and capability of your body. Such a food program emphasizes greens, good oils, and proteins (from seeds and nuts) as well as herbs and spices, both for their health benefits and deliciously wild flavors. It limits sweet and starchy foods (not too little; not too much) to the amount that your body burns as fuel in activity and emphasizes activity that builds muscle, because muscle enables you to burn carbs more effectively. A good food program strikes a balance between activity and rest and avoids toxic chemicals and drugs.

I applaud Andrew for steering you toward eating in line with nature and thinking in line with life. *Blood Sugar in Check* is easy reading, cover to cover, with helpful exercises and plans for you. Diagnosed with diabetes, you quickly begin to learn the devastating impacts of eating refined, highly processed, deep-fried, baked, and charbroiled foods. You may forget that you followed official health guidelines and feel you brought the disease on yourself. You might fear others' judgment that you're a lazy couch potato. Success in changing to a healthy lifestyle is only in part a technical issue. It also involves a shift in focus on how you feel about yourself and how you celebrate self-love and exercise self-care.

Andrew's heartfelt dedication to people with diabetes and his ability to model being vulnerable and powerful at the same time helps people with diabetes start on a new path without judgment. This makes his book a rare find. Happy reading. Happy growing. Happy thriving.

Udo Erasmus, PhD
Author of *Fats That Heal Fats That Kill*; *Omega 3 Cuisine*; and *The Book on Total Sexy Health*
Founder of *UDO'S CHOICE* supplement company, a global leader in cutting edge health products.

Advance Praise

"This book provides an easy to implement strategy for managing diabetes, yet so much more.

While of course the book is focused on thriving with diabetes, it is full of tools for the reader. The author frames the content to assist the reader out of a defeated mindset, into one of willingness to take control of their health.

There are actionable tools within the book to help the reader visually identify what areas their life needs balance. With this book, one can move out of resistance and limiting self-beliefs and into an empowered, healthy life!"

Chriss Taylor, Author of *Get The F*ck On With Your Life*

"A fearless approach to life and diabetes. Andrew Lawless is inspiring and challenging in his view on seeing diabetes as a gift. The way I think about this disease has forever changed for the better."

Kristi Brower, Author of *Relationships for Spiritual People*

If you know someone with diabetes, Blood Sugar in Check belongs in their collection of diabetes management resources. This book is judgment-free and chock full of unique tools, practical mental and physiological hacks, and inspiring stories. The science discussed in this book is relevant, easy to understand, and very well distilled. I appreciate how positive and encouraging Andrew writes throughout the book, especially when we are asked to dig deep into our minds, assessing our emotions, and behaviors. As a chronic pain relief coach and former pharmaceutical researcher, I believe that mindset and emotions affect the body's physiological equilibrium and, thus, are vital factors that affect overall health.

Everyone has a unique story and situation, but Andrew's gripping story with seemingly all odds against him is testimony that will and dedication pull us through to health and happiness with or without diabetes. If you utilize the tools and implement the strategies laid out in this book, you will be empowered to attain the satisfaction, joy, and success in your life that you deserve. Keep this book by your side and refer to it again and again. It feels like Andrew is right there cheering us on.

Eileen Paulo-Chrisco, Chief Operating Officer, *The Fascianator*[3], Author of *Pain Free Everyday*

---

[3] The Fascianator *https://www.thefascianator.com*

About This Book

My name is Andrew Lawless, and I have had type 1 diabetes since age 11. Over 40 years later, I still show no signs of complications, but some of my friends I met in the hospital when I was first diagnosed have not been so lucky. They've lost their legs eyesight, and at least one has already died from the disease. I wish I could fly back in time and give them this book; it would have made a great difference for them and their families.

Because time travel has not been invented yet, all I can do is offer this gift now. My wish for you is to live large with diabetes and, at the very least, make your life a little bit lighter, your relationship with your disease healthier, and your heart a lot warmer.

Register This Book

Please take a moment now and register this book at the link below. By doing so, I will be able to send you new insights and links to helpful articles and videos. Registration will also give you access to the free video course for this book, and you will be able to connect with peers who have diabetes.

Throughout this book, I reference worksheets that can help you gain deep insights into your Diabetes Mastery™. I have not included these forms, because formatting for the electronic and print versions of this book would not give you the best benefits from using them. But you can download them on the resource page for this book when you register it on my website today at: http://bloodsugarincheck.com.

Political Correctness

Some experts have warned me not to refer to people with diabetes as "diabetics," as many who suffer from this disease do not want to be labeled by their illness. I have tried to follow this advice as much as possible, but you will find the term all over this book, particularly when I refer to myself or include myself in the group of people with diabetes.

Why, you might ask. For me, having the label of diabetic is a badge of honor. I see more and more young people with type 1 diabetes not hiding their insulin pump anymore. This is the way it should be, and I wholeheartedly support this attitude.

This book is not for minors. It contains accounts of life experiences that are potentially difficult to read. It also uses profanity where I found it important and relevant. Be sure to read paragraphs and use your own judgment before sharing them with minors.

Typos and Grammar

Every writer knows that even after having a developmental editor, a managing editor, a line editor, and a proofreader, the moment they have their book printed, they find a major mistake in spelling, grammar, or even data.

Why would I be any different? If you do find any errors, I truly would appreciate it if you told me on the Facebook page for this book: https://www.facebook.com/groups/diabetesmentor.

Continued Conversation

Diabetes management constantly evolves with new research findings, medication, treatment options, and innovations. I wrote this book to support you in your diabetes management as these changes occur. Unless someone finds a cure for your type of diabetes, this book is designed to serve as your true companion on your way to Diabetes Mastery™.

The best way to stay informed — changes do matter, and they do happen — is to register your book as soon as you cat http://bloodsugarincheck.com.

You can also email me at andrew@bloodsugarincheck.com.

CHAPTER ONE

Stop Worrying About Dying Early from Diabetes

When we first receive the diagnosis of diabetes, we experience shock. The immediate thoughts are along the lines of *Will I lose a toe? Will my kidneys hold?* and *Will I die early?* Whatever your thoughts were when you first learned of your illness, chances are, you were focused on all the negative consequences of the disease that doctors call "the silent killer." For most of us, our attention then shifts to how to mitigate those risks and manage our diabetes to avoid the many health complications diabetes can bring.

There are disadvantages of diabetes, no doubt. But there are also advantages, as you will see. I am not trying to paint the picture better than it is. After all, diabetes is a serious disease. However, I also will not paint it worse than it is and instead shift your attention to the opportunities that diabetes gives you.

In many ways, I will reshape your inner dialogue, as well as your conversation with your diabetes health care team, so that you can lead a beautiful life with your illness. I want you to enjoy the wonders, beauty, and abundance of life. There is no reason you should hold back on your wishes and desires, deny yourself pleasures and opportunities that others take for granted, or miss out on activities, such as travel, sports, parties, hobbies, career development, or even starting your own business.

Nothing about diabetes can hold you back unless you allow it. I have never done so, and neither should you. And yes, I still have both of my kidneys and all of my toes, and my eyes have no nerve damage whatsoever. You can achieve your life dreams, not despite diabetes but because of it. When you read my story in the next chapter, you will see that if I can live a happy and meaningful life with diabetes, then you can too.

I know firsthand that the little challenges we diabetics face can derail us significantly. We have questions, self-doubts, and health concerns that most people do not even remotely think about. The most stressing one: Will my blood sugar drop at night and I'll die in bed? During waking hours, we are worried about our blood sugar dropping in client meetings, at the theater, on the beach, or in a traffic jam.

I always have sugary jelly beans with me, and for some reason, my glucose levels seem to sink most when I forget them at home and cars are moving at a stop-and-go pace. My immediate thought is *Will I make it out of here before I pass out?* Once, I even considered prying a jelly sandwich out of the hands of the kid in the car next to me. Hey, when our blood sugar drops too low, we will do anything to get food in our mouths.

We can become animals. We'll start yelling at people and become incredibly irritated about everything way before we realize what is happening to us. Once we have rebounded, we become filled with shame. I once yelled at my wife and ex-wife and made them both feel responsible for my house not being sold yet. There was nothing rational in what I said, and both of them already knew what was going on from watching me ferociously gobble jelly beans and pound apple juice. Nonetheless, I felt bad afterward. And while I was hoping that they would rationalize my behavior, which they did, the whole episode left a foul taste behind that still lingers as I write these words.

We May Win the Battle but Lose the War

On the other side of the spectrum, we have worries about long-term complications from diabetes. We have all heard stories of dogs nibbling off the toes of people with diabetes who did not feel it because their nerves had died. Diabetes can starve our nerves, make us blind, destroy our kidneys, and increase our risk for heart disease.

And as if the double whammy of worrying about dying in our sleep and losing a leg is not enough, there are day-to-day issues that can make managing our illness feel like a never-ending battle that we will ultimately lose. There is the frustration of not being able to keep blood sugar levels steady. Each time glucose spikes or bottoms out, we doubt that we will ever be healthy enough to live life, instead of just keeping on keeping on.

During these moments, the same thoughts pop up in my head: *What are my children going to do when I start fading? Will they be OK? Will they be there for me? Will I want them to have to worry about me? What about my wife? She may not have enough money to retire, and I do not want her to change my diapers or inject insulin shots into me on the regular while I am lying catatonic in bed.* My worst nightmare is being totally dependent on anyone for the most basic life tasks. I know you are, too, because you are reading this book.

There Are No Breaks

That's why I also suspect that your diabetes affects all other areas of your life as well. Going out with friends is a challenge. When is a good time to take our medication in a restaurant? How many carbs does our meal have, what's the appropriate dosage for our medication, and when and where shall we take it? Going out on a date is even trickier. When is it appropriate to tell a new friend or mate about our illness? We often worry how they will respond or react.

I have had diabetes since age 11, and at many times, especially as a teenager, I wondered if I would ever find true love. Once we enter the job world, these worries extend to our colleagues, bosses, and even clients. When is a good time to tell them? After all, we will be sitting in a lot of meetings, and sooner or later, our blood sugar will drop in one of them, and we might become irritated and unconstructive. We need people to know so that they can help us during those times, by either taking over the meeting for us or gently escorting us out to feed us orange juice before we scorch the earth.

But will they? Or will they value and respect us less because, in their minds, we have diabetes because we are fat, lazy couch potatoes whose diet consists of sugar and fat and hence we have brought the disease on ourselves?

Diabetes does not give us a break — not even when we have a break. Even a trip to the pool or beach on a hot summer day requires an incredible amount of preparation. All our friends just put on their swimsuits and get ready to jump into the water. We diabetics worry about how we will keep our blood sugar steady and whether or not our medication or insulin will overheat in our bags.

No wonder managing the disease can be overwhelming and make us depressed. Pills, pills, pills. We take pills all the time. And once we need insulin, a whole new shower of doom comes over us. We prick our fingers multiple times a day and stick needles into our bellies, legs, and butt before meals and yet still come home from a great night out or wake up in the morning with skyrocketing blood sugar levels. When does it end?

Does It End Only When We Die?

There is no doubt that diabetes needs constant attention. The older we get, the more care it needs as our bodies change and become less forgiving. So, does it end only when we die? Yes.

As an illustrative example, you may develop heart disease later in life. All types of diabetes — the latest research suggests there are five — increase your risk of heart attack, stroke, and other cardiovascular diseases exponentially with age. But context is also essential. Heart disease is a leading killer in general of both men and women. According to the Centers for Disease Control and Prevention, 610,000 people die of heart disease in the United States every year. That's about one in every four deaths of African Americans, Hispanics, Whites, American Indians, Alaska Natives, and Asians or Pacific Islanders alike.

Heart disease is everyone's problem and does not concern only people with diabetes. The principal risk factors for heart disease are high blood pressure, high cholesterol, and smoking. Eating an unhealthy diet and not getting enough exercise also increase your risk of heart disease. As a person with diabetes, you just happen to have one more risk factor.

The advantage we have as diabetics is early awareness. When you have an excellent network of doctors, your health care providers will routinely check you more thoroughly than patients without symptoms and then detect and treat issues much earlier. In contrast, many people fail to get a heart disease diagnosis soon enough. Women, for example, are sometimes labeled as having psychiatric or emotional problems or anxiety. Because of that they often receive antianxiety drugs or painkillers instead of potentially lifesaving treatments.

As a person with diabetes, your symptoms will be treated with the proper attention, sometimes even with too much care — hey, better safe than sorry. Most likely, your doctor will prescribe medication that preventively lowers blood pressure and cholesterol levels and, therefore, the risk of heart disease.

Choose to Make Your Own Luck

The other advantage of having diabetes is that by managing your disease well, you are adopting a lifestyle that reduces your risk of heart disease and many other illnesses that we commonly associate with getting old. You generally eat a healthy diet and exercise more regularly, for example — or at least you should and could.

As with everything in life, we have choices. We can focus on all the struggles, worry about the challenges we face, and infinitely seek an answer to the question, "Why me?" You and I know that such an approach is as practical as trying to fly a plane by chewing bubble gum. All it does is bring us down. We will find more evidence that gives us reason to be anxious; a bundle of nerves at our brain stem makes sure of that. It allows our brains to focus on only those pieces of information that we deem important. That's why you see more silver Toyotas on the street once you have purchased one yourself. It is also the reason you start hearing a word all the time when you've just learned it. That's where your focus is.

This bundle of nerves is called the Reticular Activating System (RAS). Now observe how often you hear that term. If you hear it more often from now on, you will have experienced the RAS in action and received a glimpse of the real impact your core beliefs and thoughts have on your life. The RAS makes you see more of what you are focused on and determines how you feel about your diabetes. Your emotions cause you to take specific actions, and your actions create results. If you believe that you are going to die early from diabetes, then you probably will. If, on the other hand, you focus on the gifts of diabetes, then your actions will lead to fulfillment in life much earlier than you would have ever achieved without the illness, and you will most likely thrive.

This is my promise to you. The purpose of this book is to shift your focus to the opportunities that diabetes brings you so that you can enjoy life again. You can manage your diabetes. You are meant to thrive. I am deeply honored that you are allowing me to be part of your amazing journey.

CHAPTER TWO

My Diabetes Life

I am writing this book because I have experienced the discrimination, humiliation, and consequences of having diabetes. I have friends who have become blind or died in their sleep. A girlfriend once dumped me because she believed my diabetes rendered me "defective." A doctor diagnosed my frozen shoulder as diabetes related when, in fact, it was the result of an untreated tendon tear.

Luckily, I have never let these things affect me and have lived life fully at every moment. But I know that living with diabetes is not easy for many, and it breaks my heart when I see people go through such an ordeal or feel ashamed, unworthy, or depressed about their illness. No one should ever have those feelings — not me, not you.

I have had type 1 diabetes for over 40 years, with no signs of long-term complications yet. I am now in a unique position to help you change your mindset so that you, too, have the fundamental tools to achieve that. I believe that how you think about yourself and your relationship with diabetes are as important as medications, what you eat, and how much you exercise.

A healthy lifestyle has nothing to do with my diabetes success; my mindset, resilience, and zest for life do. In my 20s, I used to drink a bottle of wine every night. I partied even harder. As a teenager I stayed out of the house for days and would sleep on a leather couch in a local country music bar. Privacy was not always a possibility, so I often injected insulin right through my jeans into my thigh. I rarely measured my blood sugar, and most of the time I had no idea what my glucose levels were. I just winged it.

I eventually grew up and traveled the world. I saw the pyramids of Giza from the inside, ate bushmeat in Cameroon, drove on the bombed streets of Mozambique, and tasted snakehead fish in Shanghai. I built teams for The World Bank in Moscow, Russia; Kingston, Jamaica; and Buenos Aires, Argentina.

I was unable to serve in the army when I was young, but in my 30s and 40s, I trained hostage rescue teams, Special Forces, and about 50 sheriff academies in defensive tactics and no one even knew that I have diabetes. I held top-secret security clearance and worked as a consultant to the Behavioral Science Unit of the Federal Bureau of Investigation where I supported the Global Hostage Taking Research and Analysis Program (GHost-RAP).

I have never let diabetes get in the way of my happiness, sanity, and success. And neither should you. For one, you are beautiful, marvelous, incredible, amazing, a miracle, a dream come true. Your heart started beating in your mother's womb before your brain was fully developed. What made that heart beat? Something or someone loved you enough, knew you were already enough, to give you the incredible gift of life. For as long as your heart beats, you'll live. Personal change specialist Dr. Ali Binazir equated the probability of your being born to 2.5 million people getting together to play a game of dice with a trillion-sided die and all throwing the exact same number. The odds of your coming into existence were basically zero. And yet, here you are. Life is your first gift. For me, diabetes is the second.

Life Begins with an Exorcism

Caution: My managing editor advised me, "Without minimizing the seriousness and importance of those early experiences, could you warn the reader at the start of this section that you'll be sharing some potentially difficult to read life experiences?" I do not see it that way, because when we blame life for our pains and injustices, we also need to thank it for shaping us into the people we are today. However, I am coachable. So, here you go: Potentially difficult-to-read life experiences ahead.

I was diagnosed with type 1 diabetes when I was 11 years old.

That's when the beatings stopped at home. It may be the reason I have always looked at the illness as a blessing. My childhood was pretty shitty until my diagnosis. I have no active memory of my childhood, apart from the pain and injuries. The rest I only know from stories other people have told me. My life began when I was diagnosed with diabetes.

I was born out of wedlock, and in 1965 it was hard luck in Germany for an unmarried woman to have a child. My mother was not even able to find anyone who would baptize me, until she convinced a Catholic priest to do it, but she had to agree to his condition that he also perform an exorcism on me. That's why I am the only Catholic in the entire family. It also shaped my relationship with organized religion. To this day, I joke that my whole life unfolds from there: exorcism.

At age 3 I almost died in a freak accident when a steel gate pulled and squished me into a retracting wall. The injuries were so severe that doctors considered amputating my left leg but ultimately decided against it. Today, I still walk with a limp, my ribs stick out funny, and my eyes are not on the same axis on my face. Until age 10, I was only able to walk up stairs one at a time, which made me a natural target for bullies. And there were many of them.

I grew up in Düsseldorf-Gerresheim, Germany, in a blue-collar area next to a glass factory, with railroad tracks in between. It was the kind of neighborhood that could be the backdrop of a Bruce Springsteen song. Law enforcement officers would not get out of their cars, and when you saw a red light, you would not stop.

Limping and unable to run, I would get beaten up fairly regularly. There was a small bridge over the river Düssel that I needed to cross on my way to school, and every morning and afternoon, boys would wait for me to give me a beating. One day they raped me. Another time at school, someone unhinged a steel door and pushed it onto me, causing one of the hinges to puncture a hole in the back of my head.

But the worst part was coming home, where the beatings continued. One day, I tore my sheepskin leather jacket when the bridge boys pushed me into the bushes. When I came home afterward, my mother beat me with the heels of her shoes as a punishment. On other days, she used wooden spoons, her hands, or whatever was available. Her philosophy of learning was, and I quote, "Beatings to the back of the head increase your ability to think."

It worked for a while. I was a good student in elementary school and graduated to Gymnasium, which in Germany was the only educational track that allowed a student to go to college or university. But in sixth grade, I suddenly went from all *As* to all *Fs*, which prevented me from advancing to seventh grade. My performance was so bad that the principal even put a remark on my report card that I was suitable only for special education, which would have prevented me from ever getting a decent job.

My Second Gift in Life: Diabetes

I had not suddenly lost my marbles. It turned out that I had developed diabetes and wandered around in a half coma for almost a year. All I would do at home was lie on the couch and stare at the ceiling. I remember drinking a lot of *Coca-Cola* and needing to pee all the time, but no one was really concerned until my older stepbrother learned about diabetes in biology class. My mother took me to the doctor's office, and I was diagnosed with type 1.

At the time, I did not fully grasp what having diabetes meant or how permanent and potentially deadly the disease is. For all I knew, diabetes was a blessing, because my mother became less violent. My suspicion is that she blamed herself for my having diabetes, but we never talked about it.

Inside and outside of school, I was now always under close supervision, so the bridge boys left me alone most of the time. For me, diabetes meant relief. I still feel that way today. My hypnotist, Tatiana Watson (look her up if you live in the Washington, DC area), firmly believes that my body developed diabetes to protect me. That may sound like a far-fetched idea, but scientists have confirmed that "experience of a serious life event (reasonably indicating psychological stress) during the first 14 years of life may be a risk factor for [developing] type 1 diabetes."

Be that as it may, diabetes enabled me to shift my attention from the scary to the enlightening. I did not get sucked into the drug scene like my older stepbrother and instead filled my brain with the teachings of major philosophies, such as Taoism, Buddhism, and Hinduism. Lao-tzu, Buddha, and Alan Watts became my teachers. Diabetes can be incredibly rewarding when we look in the right places.

At the time, doctors did not want us type 1 diabetics to do a lot of sports out of concern that our blood sugar could drop and possibly cause us to pass out. Insulin pens had just emerged on the market, and I injected pig-derived insulin twice daily but largely managed my blood sugar through food intake. That did not fly well with me. I wanted to be a professional athlete and to support five to six hours of daily training, I figured out a methodology to eat about 7,000 calories per day, keep my blood sugar within a healthy range, and become one of Germany's top 10 Frisbee players. You can still read the article here if you understand German.

But I tore the meniscus on my right knee during a German Ultimate Frisbee Championship match and subsequently traded the disc for a Commodore C64 home computer and educated myself on how to use and program it. Germany's leading computer magazine was looking for editors who could reach a mainstream audience; the fact that I had basic programming skills and a published article qualified me for the job.

A year later I wrote a beginner's guide to the Commodore C64 (you can read it here, also in German), which became the number one best-selling computer book for 11 months. That success, in turn, prompted an editor for the German edition of Forbes magazine to have me exclusively interview Bill Gates at Frankfurt Airport. Bill was on his way to Moscow to introduce the Cyrillic version of MS-DOS 4.0, and no other available journalist in Germany knew how important that was.

With a cover story in *Forbes* magazine, my career skyrocketed. I eventually worked alongside the owner of Germany's second-largest publishing group at the time. Dr. Stefan von Holtzbrinck, of *Holtzbrinck Publishing Group*, sent me to work out of *Scientific American's* offices in New York, NY, and sponsored my green card.

After that gig, I drove a corporate turnaround at *Berlitz* in Central and Eastern Europe and transformed the way *The World Bank* manages worldwide translation and interpretation services to this day. I am now a diabetes coach and use tools and methodologies from *Strategic Intervention* that have helped my executive clients and small business owners thrive. I learned and developed some of the tools and strategies in this book when I was a consultant to the Behavioral Science Unit of the Federal Bureau of Investigation in Quantico, Virginia. As of this writing, I have just been nominated as a finalist for the prestigious 2018 Kolbe Professional Award in recognition of my changing many lives.

My Third Gift

I am not sharing this success with you to impress you but to impress upon you that you can do anything you'd like with diabetes if you learn to see the possibilities and the gifts it brings. When we blame the people and circumstances in our lives, we also need to thank them for the gifts they brought us. Would I ever have left my rough neighborhood in Germany and immigrated to the United States if my childhood had been more protected? Would I have picked up a Commodore C64 home computer, which led to an interview with Bill Gates? And would I be able to write this book and have the opportunity to change your life if I had not had to get my own life in order first?

You are my third gift. I have the unique opportunity to contribute to your living life the way you want and deserve. Before this book existed, it was just an idea. Only my focus on writing made it a book. But you alone give it value. You deeply honor me by reading this book, and I thank you from the bottom of my heart for this remarkable honor.

And always remember, it all started with an exorcism.

CHAPTER THREE

The Diabetes Mastery™ Process

The first step to getting your blood sugar in check is to differentiate the technical issues of managing your illness from the behavioral challenges of enabling yourself to live a healthy and fulfilling life. Most illnesses can be treated through diagnosis and treatment. When you have a cold, you can typically ease your symptoms with over-the-counter medications, and after a few days or couple of weeks, you are back to normal. Treating a cold is a technical problem. Even measles, a once deadly and still highly contagious virus that grows in cells in the lungs and can lead to pneumonia, is by and large treatable. Appendicitis, which was also deadly at one time, can be cured by routine surgery or antibiotics. Tuberculosis is entirely curable today by taking antibiotics for 6 to 9 months.

Treating a cold, appendicitis, or tuberculosis is a technical issue. It is not trivial though. A doctor still needs to diagnose the illness and determine the appropriate therapy plan. Developing medication for these diseases is very complex. Finding cures took decades, if not centuries, to develop. Even today, it takes 10 years or longer for a new medicine to make it to the marketplace, and the average cost to develop a drug is about $2.6 billion. What makes the diagnose-and-treat method a technical issue is that there are established processes in place to detect a curable illness and then prescribe medication or perform surgery or a procedure to end it.

Treating Diabetes Is Technically Easy

Diabetes is different from curable diseases because there is no cure. Yes, many promising medical trials suggest we may soon get healed entirely. It is also true that I have heard that news for over 40 years and a cure is still not available to me.

For now, your best bet is to successfully treat the symptoms of diabetes, which on the most basic level means keeping your glucose levels within the following ranges:

- Between 80 and 100 mg/dl (5.6 mmol/L) before a meal

- Below 160 mg/dl (8.9 mmol/L) 2 hours after a meal

- Below 126 mg/dl (7.0 mmol/L) over a period of 3 months on average

Please note that in the US and Germany, which are my countries of reference, people measure blood sugar–level concentration in milligrams per deciliter (mg/dL). I will use these measurements throughout this book, even though the international standard is to measure glucose in your blood in terms of molar concentration, measured in millimoles per liter (mmol/L). You can find many resources on the Internet with tables that show mmol/L to mg/dl conversions, with some including printable charts. Just search for "mmol/L to mg/dL conversion". Personally, I use the *Blood Sugar* app from the *App Store*.

To achieve these goals, just follow these five rules:

1. Measure blood sugar 5–7 times a day (if you do not have an insulin pump that does the job for you).

2. Keep glucose levels in check by taking your medication as prescribed.

3. Practice yoga or walk for at least 30 minutes every day.

4. Stay hydrated.

5. Follow an alkaline diet.

It is that easy, until you realize that an alkaline diet includes avoiding all foods that are white, such as sugar, potatoes, rice, noodles, cheese, yogurt, milk, and bread. You are not allowed to eat beef or chicken either or drink alcohol or caffeine. Canned and packaged snacks as well as fast foods, are off the table. You are left with eating water-based fruits and vegetables, soybeans and tofu, and some nuts, seeds, legumes, and essential fats.

You may wonder if such a diet is practical or even entirely healthy. Every body is different and has its own unique needs. I am using the example of an alkaline diet because I have recently started to follow it with remarkable results. Your diabetes care team may suggest a different diet for you, and it will most likely also restrict what or how much you can eat in some fashion that you won't like.

When it comes to the extreme alkaline diet, I can almost hear your lack of enthusiasm about it:

- "I hate the idea of that diet. I cannot live without bread, meat, and potatoes."

- "I cannot function without my cup of java in the morning."

- "I need that glass of red wine to relax at home after a hard day of work."

- "It is impossible to fit 30 minutes of exercise into my everyday routine."

- "I cannot maintain my diabetes routines when I travel or eat out."

These excuses are what we call a behavioral challenge.

Managing Diabetes Requires You to
Change Your Behavior

Maintaining a healthy weight is vital in treating diabetes and preventing long-term complications. An alkaline diet, for example, helps you reach your target weight quickly and keep the pounds off. It also helps lower blood pressure and cholesterol, the two significant risk factors for heart disease. That's super important for people with diabetes.

According to the American Heart Association, "at least 68% of people age 65 or older with diabetes die from some form of heart disease; and 16% die of stroke. Adults with diabetes are two to four times more likely to die from heart disease than adults without diabetes." And yet, many diabetics want to go back to the life they know rather than adopt a lifestyle that ensures they will be around long enough to support their children, grandchildren, and loved ones without being a burden to them. They'd rather give up a happy retirement in excellent health in favor of meat and potatoes and choose the likelihood of losing the ability to move their left arm, speak, or hold their pee – all typical side effects of a stroke—than change what they eat. How does that make sense?

Behavioral change is hard and takes time. There are basic needs, fears, and forces that pull us in opposite directions all the time. We know that we will need to change our diet, for example, but we only see results after a few weeks, months, or even years.

On the other hand, there are cold beers, bratwursts, and fries available right there at the BBQ, or sugar cookies at a school event, or that cheese board at a friend's birthday party.

Your behavioral challenges do not end with the food you put in your mouth. They continue through all facets of your life. You will need to bring your medication to the pool and make sure it won't overheat. You will need to plan your business meeting with a client so that your blood sugar won't drop low during your presentation. Traveling internationally will require you to prepare your body clock for the time zone change differently than you have done before. You will need to spill the beans about your diabetes to a new friend, colleague, or boss. Even your new yoga teacher and fitness class trainer will need to know, even though you do not trust them yet. But they will ask why you brought jelly beans to class.

Your 7 Step Diabetes Mastery™ Process

At this very moment, you may not be sure if you will ever be able to make the changes that will keep your blood sugar in check. Relax, because, yes, you will. I have broken down your transformation into an easy Diabetes Mastery™ Process with seven steps.

I am also not suggesting that you must follow a strict alkaline diet. After all, even the American Heart Association has guacamole, deviled eggs, and beef stew on their list of healthy recipes. You can zigzag. Perfection is the enemy of execution, and I'd rather you do it 80% right than not at all. As long as you keep on moving forward toward your goals, you are heading in the right direction.

In the following chapters, I will share with you a process to make the successful transformation to a healthy and rewarding life with diabetes, free from guilt and anxiety. I will show you the seven steps of the Diabetes Mastery™ Process that hundreds of my coaching clients have successfully taken to make significant life changes. They have used the same process to save their businesses, repair their relationships, find their dream jobs, or advance their careers—and of course live happy and healthy lives.

The seven steps are:

Step 1: Understand what's holding you back. You will understand why knowing which changes you want to make to manage your diabetes is easy but following through is hard. I will introduce you to common mental roadblocks and how you can use your mind to thrive and succeed in your diabetes care.

Step 2: Create your Wheel of Diabetes Mastery™. In this step, we will get real and paint a picture of where you stand in all aspects of your life that impact your ability to manage your blood sugar. With a very effective exercise, I will help you narrow your focus to the one life area that you will need to work on for a positive impact on your overall diabetes success.

Step 3: Design your personal diabetes plan. At the end of this chapter, you will understand why you are not getting positive results in your current diabetes management. I will help you understand the natural talents that define what you will and won't naturally do to get your blood sugar in check. You will begin to design your personal diabetes plan based on the strengths that are already in you.

Step 4: Find your diabetes flow. Here, you will find which diabetes management tasks will give you the most value and benefits. You will identify techniques that stress you out and then dump them so you can focus on practices that you like and can follow with ease.

Step 5: Condition yourself for blood sugar success. At the end of this chapter, you will begin developing a new relationship with diabetes by incorporating new insights about yourself and your feelings about your illness. You will begin to talk and think differently and change the way you feel about keeping your blood sugar in check.

Step 6: Overcome unconstructive blood sugar management patterns. In this step, you will make your personalized, healthy routines a lifelong habit. I will help you find behavioral patterns that have sabotaged your diabetes management in the past and then identify new routines that support your blood sugar goals.

Step 7: Embrace your diabetes lifestyle. You will finish your transformation in this section by eliminating unconstructive behaviors and replacing them with concrete to-dos that help you achieve lasting and continuous life success with diabetes.

At the end of this section, I listed a few practical hacks that I have found useful in my own diabetes management from keeping insulin cool when I travel to using smart phones to help me keep my blood sugar in check at home. I will talk about potential obstacles that can blindside you and how you can avoid them.

When you have finished reading, and after you have completed all the exercises, you will be able to develop your own way of managing your life with diabetes. You will do it in a way that works for you, keeps you energized, and nourishes your zest for life. A good sign is if at the end you are excited and inspired by this book but also feel a bit scared or uncomfortable. This typically means that you are stimulated to grow and ready to commit to progress.

Let's begin the journey!

CHAPTER FOUR

Step 1: Understand What's Holding You Back

Most people give up on their New Year's resolutions by the end of January – within just three weeks. The same thing happens to people with diabetes. Shortly after diagnosis they are determined to have their A1c in range, exercise regularly, eat healthy, measure their blood sugar multiple times a day, take their medication religiously, keep a journal, and so on.

Once the honeymoon with diabetes comes to a close, their illness brings about emotions and realizations that this is their new life forever and it can be very daunting at times. Managing the day to day is much harder and takes much more time than expected. As a result, they often fall back into old habits that they like but are no longer beneficial to them, like eating pizza or drinking too much wine.

Knowing which changes to make is easy but following through on them is hard. The mind plays clever tricks on you, and unless you outsmart it, your brain wins.

Your Brain Is Made for Survival,
Not Blood Sugar Success

As human beings, we are not the fastest or strongest species on Earth, yet we dominate the planet. New studies suggest that our ancestors' bodies began rerouting energy flow from the muscles to the brain when modern humans and chimps diverged about 6 million years ago. That's why today even an untrained chimp will beat university-level basketball players in weight lifting.

With this evolution, the responsibility for survival moved from muscle to brain. The human brain's primary function is not to make us creative, or happy, or confident. The opposite is true. It is to keep us alive, and thus, the brain is also is the master of bringing to our attention everything around us that could be a danger. Our brains and our bodies are made for survival.

That served us well 10,000 years ago, when it was important for us to detect the lioness that wants to eat us behind the bush, learn that bitter fruits can poison us, detect patterns in clouds that project incoming severe weather, interpret ill intentions in a person's face, and so on.

Back then, most changes in our lives were bad news. They were mostly a threat to our survival, and the human brain helped us figure out multiple ways of detecting and mitigating risks. We figured out how to grow, cook, preserve, and store food to survive the change from warmth in summer to cold during winter. In the process, we developed eating habits, lifestyles, and social behavior that helped us endure and survive then but no longer serve us diabetics now. They may even be the reason we developed diabetes in the first place.

But the brain does not change that fast. It has not even adjusted to the way we have communicated and lived with technology in the past 50 years. So do not expect it to change overnight with your diabetes. It took millions of years for the brain to function like it does today and to put systems in place to help us survive.

The brain releases hormones, such as endorphins, that make the pain go away. Our bodies evolved a dopamine system that differs from the ones in chimpanzees to keep us motivated and focused on getting food. Cortisol makes us alert to danger. Adrenaline opens the lungs' airways and helps increase blood flow and blood pressure to bring oxygen and energy to our muscles to fight, flight, or freeze out of a dangerous situation.

The human body can go into survival mode and endure extreme temperatures for weeks without food. As long as a person drinks water, he or she can live up to 8 weeks without food. The Dutch extreme athlete Wim Hof, also known as The Iceman, has shown that with the right breathing alone, he can climb Mount Everest wearing only shorts and shoes—no shirt, jacket, or oxygen mask. He has also run a full marathon in the Namib Desert without water.

We are made for endurance and survival, and we can strengthen that ability by conditioning our bodies and minds. In fact, we do that all the time (maybe not to climb Mount Everest in shorts but to endure everyday situations and circumstances). That's the reason people stay in lousy jobs or crappy relationships much longer than they should. I know that you have, too, at one point in your life. That's when the survival mechanism works against you.

Two Basic Fears That Sabotage
Your Diabetes Management

We are made to endure, not change. In fact, our brains will actively fight us when we want to change to routines that support our diabetes health.

Take, for example, weight loss. There are two forces in our heads that pull us in opposite directions. On one side, there is the desire to relieve the pain of feeling too heavy by losing weight. But there is always food and a glass of wine available when we need instant relaxation after a hard day at work.

The internal struggle exists between avoiding pain and gaining pleasure. Your brain will want you to survive in the short term, causing long-term goals to fall by the wayside. It can take months before we see decent weight loss results, but the benefits and pleasures of eating are instant.

The brain wants us to eat and have that glass of wine. It wants us to be fat. Science confirms that the brain actively fights back when we diet. It makes neurological changes so that food gives us a bigger rush of the reward hormone dopamine. That's the same hormone that is released when addicts use their drug of choice.

But that's not all. With our bodies and a meal plan, our brains also lower levels of leptin, a hormone that decreases appetite, while elevating levels of ghrelin, a hormone that increases appetite.

Talk about an aggressive defense on three fronts. The brain changes levels of dopamine, leptin, and ghrelin to make us eat more than we want and should. It goes into hormonal overdrive because it wants to protect us. As weird as this may sound, our bodies need us to eat so that they can store fat to survive. Fat not only helps us pull through famine but also ensures that our blood, organs, glands, and tissues remain slightly alkaline.

The body cannot live when it is acidic. It needs to remain slightly alkaline to maintain health. One way for the brain to reduce acidity is to store it in fat cells. That's why many commercial diet programs don't work long term.

Packaged, prepared, and processed meals may help us lose weight temporarily, because we are consuming fewer calories than we need. But because the body has less fat available when we have completed the program, it tends to become more acidic, which is why many people experience a lack of energy while on a diet plan. Once the diet is over, we often regain energy and a zest for life. We also start adding weight again, because the body goes into alkalizing overdrive and rushes to store acids in our fat cells. So, the brain gets what it wants the body to have and thus succeeds in undermining what the mind-set is out to achieve.

Our brains actively sabotage us when we diet and when we want to give up smoking or drinking, go to the gym, or begin introducing new diabetes management routines. Whatever we want to change, the human brain will initially interpret it as a threat, and in many ways it believes that you, personally, are the greatest risk to survival. After all, it's you who initiates change.

Your Mind Will Need to Wrestle
Your Brain into Diabetes Management

Stanford University professor Alia Crum proved how our mind-sets matter in virtually every facet of our lives, health, and well-being. She found that the mind affects how the brain releases hormones into the body much more than we think.

Having exercised for 4 hours every day, she began asking herself one critical question: Was she getting fitter and stronger because of the time and energy she put into her training or merely that she believed she would? She also asked herself if people who get the same amount of exercise without being aware of it would get the same amount of health benefits.

She found her answer by working with 48 housekeepers in 7 different hotels across the United States. Because their work is physical, housekeepers burn between 160 and 240 calories an hour. Yet most of them do not see their work as exercise.

Crum split the women into two groups. The first was told their work did not equal a healthy workout. She gave the second group a different message. With a 15-minute, convincing presentation, she told them they could expect multiple health benefits from just doing their jobs.

Four weeks later, she found that the latter group had lost a significant amount of weight and body fat and had lower blood pressure. The women in group 2 also reported higher job satisfaction. At the same time, there was no change in the first group of women, who kept their old mind-set.

Crum changed the whole game for 24 women with just a simple 15-minute presentation that altered the way they viewed their work. This is exactly what you are going to do in the remainder of this book. You will create a mind-set that supports you in improving your blood sugar levels and overall health.

Perception Is Reality – Your Hormones Agree

It's not voodoo science. You may believe that this is wishful thinking and that weight loss is one thing, but managing your hormones, such as insulin, is quite another. And Crum thought so too. She wanted to know if this experiment was replicable in a different environment and if it zeroed in on hormones.

Crum scheduled her students for two 2.5-hour sessions at the Yale Clinical Center for Investigation Hospital Research Unit to test two different kinds of milkshakes. In the first week, the students drank a "sensible" low-calorie, low-fat version; in the second week, the same students drank a high-fat, high-calorie "indulgent" shake. She shared that the sensible shake contained 140 calories and the indulgent version contained 620 calories.

What the students did not know is that both shakes were identical in nutrients: 13 grams of fat, 47 carbohydrates, and 380 calories. Crum wanted to know if just reading and believing different nutrition labels would change the levels of the hunger hormone ghrelin.

When we have not eaten for a while, ghrelin in our guts rises and tells us to seek out food, and causes the slowing of our metabolism just in case we don't find it soon. Once we have eaten plenty of calorie-laden food, our ghrelin levels drop and our metabolism increases, signaling that it is time to stop eating. Ghrelin levels drop in proportion to the calories consumed. The more calories we put into our bodies, the more ghrelin levels drop.

To measure the ghrelin response, Crum's team placed an intravenous catheter in each participant at each milkshake session. The results are a stunning testimony to the power of the mind. Ghrelin levels dropped three times more in participants who believed they'd drunk the decadent milkshake compared with those who thought they'd drunk the sensible version.

Remember, they consumed the same milkshake each time; nonetheless, they felt full after drinking the one they believed had more calories, fat, and protein, and were still hungry after drinking what they thought was the low-calorie version.

If a simple nutrition label can mind-wrestle your autonomous nervous system, then imagine what life could be like if you conditioned your brain to believe that you manage your diabetes well and that you have all the energy in the world to thrive with your illness. What if you overcame the fear of being too busy, too active, too skinny, too fat, too worried, too depressed, too disorganized, or too disadvantaged to manage your diabetes?

Whatever you are telling yourself will come true. You can stop being hungry just by believing that you have consumed a tremendous number of calories, even if you have not. Your blood pressure can drop just by thinking your job meets the criteria for a healthy lifestyle.

Is it then possible that your blood sugar increases just because you are telling yourself that you are not good enough or even incapable of getting it under control? Research is limited for diabetes, but what is available has shown that anxiety increases blood glucose levels quickly and substantially. If you struggle with managing your diabetes, perhaps it's because you do everything right, but how you feel about yourself and your level of anxiety make it impossible to get your blood sugar levels in check. It's all in your head.

Conquer Your Two Basic Diabetes Fears

There are two stories that we make up in our minds all the time that alert us to the dangers of diabetes. When you first learned about your illness, your brain went into survival mode and warned you of everything that could possibly harm you. The most obvious danger was that you may not be good enough to handle your disease. The second danger it noticed was that if you failed to keep your blood sugar in check, then you would lose your ability to function in your job, family, and social life and may no longer be respected, liked, or loved as a result.

Fear 1: "I'm not good enough for this diabetes thing."

No matter how successful you may be, the fear of not being good enough is present in almost all aspects of your life whenever you want to do something new. Diabetes is just one of them. I had lunch earlier this year with a self-made billionaire, who revealed to me that her biggest concern was not being good enough to follow her heart and start a business in an entirely new field. Here is a woman who has achieved more than most of us dream of and still doubts that she is good enough.

When first diagnosed, most people with diabetes share the

same fear. They struggle with leading a new life because they do not want to be perceived as a failure or beginner. That's particularly true when they are accomplished in their careers. It takes a special person and mind-set to become a student again after having achieved status in our jobs and lives. At a point where we are perceived as experts in our fields, when we have developed and fostered relationships with friends, family, colleagues, and clients, and after we have received recognition for our accomplishments, who wants to be a failure?

Changing our diet and exercise habits, adding routines to measure blood sugar, and counting carbohydrates is hard. It requires us to start over. Being a beginner again makes us anxious, and these emotions lead us to resist change. The fear of not being good enough paralyzes us. Fear is often a stronger force than willpower.

Most people want a guarantee that their efforts will bear fruit, but that's not how it works. Change and growth take place in sustained periods of discomfort. The reality is that your blood sugar will never again be perfect most of the time. Sometimes you will come home from a dinner party with your glucose levels skyrocketing. At other times, it will be super low. You will have days where your numbers jump up and down no matter what you do, and you'll struggle to get them back in balance.

Fear 2: "People will judge me for having diabetes."

You will have business meetings where you need to step out and get your blood sugar back up. Your significant other or friends will hear your slurred speech or be taken aback by your aggressiveness when your blood sugar sinks below a certain point. The people around you will learn to see and interpret the signs of hypoglycemia before you do, and they will give you space as well as encouragement to take care of yourself. They will forgive your behavior. And if they don't, and you feel hurt, then recognize this emotion as a signal that you have expectations that cannot be met. It's a call for you to change your perception, way of communicating your needs, or behavior, or to surround yourself with better people.

Remember that success is a result of making sound judgments, which in turn come from experience. And experience often comes from failure, which is a result of bad judgment. So, whenever your numbers are not perfect, which will be most of the time, you are one step closer to your goal of managing your diabetes well. Every high or low is your reminder that you must learn and take new action.

Someone once calculated that the mountaineer Reinhold Messner has had a 99.9% chance of being killed on his expeditions. Yet he was the first person to climb Mount Everest alone, the first to climb all 14 eight-thousanders, and the fifth to finish the Seven Summits. He is a living legend among climbers.

When he initially proposed climbing Everest without oxygen, in 1978, people told him it was not possible and that he was risking his life. They said he would lose his brains up there. Indeed, uncertainty, failure, and hard work filled his path to success. After his two first expeditions to the Himalayas, he lost three teammates, including his brother Günther. He failed on several other expeditions in the '70s. But that did not stop him.

When he made his first solo climb without oxygen, in 1980, Messner described himself as "nothing more than a single narrow gasping lung" as he summited Everest. "Climbing Everest solo without bottled oxygen in 1980 was the hardest thing I've done. I was alone up there, completely alone. I fell down a crevasse at night and almost gave up," he told Observer Magazine.

Messner says he always takes the same perspective with each new adventure. In his own words, "I put myself in the position of being at the end of my life looking back. Then I ask myself if what I am doing is important to me. [...] Failing is more important than having success."

Managing diabetes may be your mountain to climb. Do not let your fear of being judged allow you to stop moving up. All your emotions around diabetes are a call to action. Apprehension is a signal to prepare or get prepared to deal with something that is about to come. Anticipate and adjust. If it is beyond your control, then change your perception and let it go.

I also know that this is easier said than done, especially during times when we do fail. When I yelled at both my current and ex-wife during a low–blood sugar episode, I felt terrible afterward. First, guilt crept in. I deeply regretted my actions because I'd violated one of my own standards. I have learned not to stay in guilt, but I also do not deny it and make things right when I screw up. The people who love us, the ones who are worth holding onto, will easily rationalize our behavior. I am sure you, too, justified the behavior of a loved one in the past yourself.

The two basic fears play mind tricks on you. Therefore, you will need to mind-wrestle your brain through a sustained period of discomfort. There is no guarantee that what you are doing is going to work, but don't be disappointed. Realize that an expectation or desired outcome may not happen and that you'll need to change your expectation. For example, maybe your time frame for getting your A1c down was too short, and you'll need to extend it going forward.

The Two Forces That Drive Our Diabetes Routines

There are two behavioral forces that can help you manage your diabetes without the fears of not being good enough to manage your diabetes and being judged if you fail to do so. Whenever fears hold you back, these two forces can pull you into a healthy direction when you align them. One force is the need to avoid pain; the other is the desire to gain pleasure.

To understand how these two forces work, I use weight loss as an example again. It is one of the most significant challenges for people with diabetes, so it serves as the handiest case study. No one actually wants to have to lose weight. Most people do not enjoy going on a diet, even a tiny bit. Diets are painful. They require you to introduce a lot of change into your life, such as what you eat, how much you eat, what you cannot eat, how to cook differently, and so on. You will need to buy different foods, try new recipes, and acquire a taste for new spices, tofu, or chickpeas. That's a lot of change.

There can only be one explanation for why people voluntarily subject themselves to that kind of ordeal. The pain associated with being overweight must be more significant than the anticipated pain that comes with a diet.

The pain, however, can be varied. Maybe they hate the way they look. Perhaps they cannot walk up the stairs without huffing and coughing and getting out of breath. As a person with diabetes, they will worry about all the long-term health consequences, such as sleep apnea, cancer, or dying early from a stroke.

In my case, it was a blockage in one of my arteries from my martial arts days, when I would devour porterhouse steaks and eggs to pump protein into my muscles. Luckily, the blockage did not inhibit blood flow, so I did not need a stent, but my cardiologists told me that it was just a matter of time, mainly because I am a diabetic. They all recommended a vegan diet, which could slow down the process, if not completely reverse the blockage.

That's not a message any meat lover wants to hear. At the time, a great summer Saturday night on my patio included a juicy steak and a few glasses of red wine. But I could not stand the thought of not being actively involved in my then 6-year-old son's upbringing—or, even worse, not being around for long. So, I became a vegan, cold turkey, no pun intended.

I have not gone back to eating meat since. The trick was to make the journey fun, meaningful, and pleasurable. In support of me, my wife turned vegan herself, and we experimented with trying new recipes, tasting new food, finding different restaurants, going to yoga classes, inviting new friends into our lives who are vegan, and so on. We even laughed hard when we heard each other fart while our digestive systems changed, knowing that with each fart, we were one step closer to our goal.

We were also aware that a desire for perfection is the enemy of progress. Being strictly vegan is not an option when we travel. It is hard to find vegan options, let alone alkaline ones, at an airport. Most food in restaurants, convenience stores, and conferences are either meat based or full of empty carbohydrates. So, we learned not to be too hard on ourselves and to switch to a vegetarian diet as we traveled, and enjoy, rather than regret, eating that cheese sandwich.

However, the need to avoid pain and the desire to gain

pleasure do not always pull in the same direction. On one hand, my goal was to reverse the blockage in my heart. On the other hand, it takes years to achieve this goal. Progress is also hard to measure, and it ultimately requires a cardiac catheterization to validate improvement, if any. At the same time, delicious chocolates and fully loaded ice cream sundaes are always available and give instant pleasure. In the beginning, I gave into those treats too much and too often.

When the two forces that drive our behavior pull in different directions, something very interesting and unhealthy happens. At first, I got a total emotional high from the delicious ice cream. Then, the next day or even an hour later, I'd regret my decision. Ice cream is full of ingredients I am not supposed to eat, such as milk, sugar, fat, and more sugar. Each time that happened, I realized that I had sabotaged my goal of reversing the heart blockage. I felt like a failure and was depressed for a while, until I snapped out of it with the determination to never, ever eat ice cream again. And then, a few days or weeks later, I would go out with my youngest son for dinner and, sure enough, indulge in ice cream again.

And so began the whole roller coaster ride of emotions, from joy to depression and back again ... and again ... and again. Like Groundhog Day. What I needed to do was align my need to avoid complications with my desire to enjoy food.

Any progress you want to make requires you to conquer the fear of not being good enough and align your need to avoid pain with your desire to gain pleasure. This is the first step in your diabetes transformation process, because it is the condition for you to stick with your diabetes health plan. Without these alignments, you will revert to what you have done in the past without positive results. If you have ever made plans to lose weight, save money, go to the gym every day, or read a new book each week and did not maintain momentum, then the same will happen with your plans for Diabetes Mastery™.

That is why I let you finish this chapter by beginning a process to align your driving behavioral forces.

Going Away Things

In this process, you will first list everything in your life that stands in your way. Use the worksheet called "Going-Away Things," which you can find in my Facebook group or download the files from the resource website for this book at http://BloodSugarInCheck.com. You also can just take a blank sheet of paper, draw a line from top to bottom, and only use the left column for this exercise.

Now list in the left column all the things in your life with diabetes that you want to disappear. We call them the going-away things, which comprise everything that causes you depression, boredom, being overwhelmed, anger, worry, frustration, resentment, sadness, jealousy, self-pity, hurt, guilt, and feelings of being inadequate, overloaded, or lonely.

Only write in the left column and leave the right one empty for now. If you run out of space, continue on a second copy of this worksheet. You will fill in the lines on the right column shortly and will need that empty space on the right further down in this chapter.

Make sure no one disturbs you and nothing distracts you during this exercise. Turn off everything that can divert your attention while you write. Turn off your notifications on your laptop, phone, tablet, smart watch, smart speakers, and anything else that can give you an alert. You are about to discover new insights and strategies. You deserve this time.

Do not continue reading this book until you have completed this exercise. The rest of this book relies on the outcome of the alignment of your behavioral forces. You will benefit from reading the following chapters without completing your list of going-away things, but you will only be able to take full advantage of all the strategies when you have written your thoughts down.

So, start writing now.

When you are done, your list may look like this:

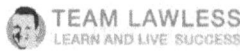

TEAM LAWLESS
LEARN AND LIVE SUCCESS

Going-Away Things

Everything that causes me depression, boredom, being overwhelmed, anger, worry, frustration, resentment, sadness, jealousy, self-pity

Going-Away Things

Going-Away Things	
My weight	
Hypos at night	
Extreme high blood sugar after breakfast	
Restrictive diet	
Insulin shots and needles	
Daily stress of managing my diabetes	
Low sex drive	
My mood swings	
Worry over long-term complications	
Fear of leaving the house alone	
Stomach problems	
My unsupportive spouse	

Your next step is to list in the right column all the reasons that have kept you from resolving the issue. You'll write down next to each going-away thing why it is still there. They are on your list because you would have not mentioned them here if you had already addressed them.

Something important, fearful, or unusual is still going on that you have not resolved yet. You may even have put it off because it is too stressful for you to think about, and you try not to focus on it. Or maybe you are practicing positive thinking and hoping these issues will eventually go away by themselves or somehow get magically resolved otherwise.

Your challenges will not disappear until you make them go away. I am all for positive thinking, but thoughts without action are wasted. Only positive action will bring a change. And we will start by addressing them head-on.

Start writing now.

When you are done, your list may now look like this:

Going-Away Things

Everything that causes me depression, boredom, being overwhelmed, anger, worry, frustration, resentment, sadness, jealousy, self-pity

Going-Away Things

My weight	I cannot live without bread, pasta, and wine.
Hypos at night	I need a few glasses of wine at night to calm me down.
Extreme high blood sugar after breakfast	I cannot give up granola and orange juice in the morning.
Restrictive diet	I hate a plant-based diet. My body needs animal protein.
Insulin shots and needles	I am afraid of needles.
Daily stress of managing my diabetes	I won't be able to handle the lifelong diabetes management thing. It's too much.
Low sex drive	Because of my diabetes, I am just not that aroused anymore.
My mood swings	My life with diabetes is always on my mind. I cannot be chipper.
Worry over long-term complications	I will never be good at managing my diabetes It's just a matter of time.
Fear of leaving the house alone	No one will help me when I am alone and I need quick help to get my blood sugar back up .
Stomach problems	I cannot give up white bread, pasta, and rice, and granola bars.

I applaud you for being honest with yourself. The one person we lie to the most is ourselves. And this time, you kept yourself real. You have now successfully created clarity in your head about what holds you back. From now on, you will call these reasons your limiting beliefs. These are incorrect conclusions about yourself and your diabetes that keep you from succeeding.

Your last task is to write the headline "Limiting Beliefs" in red on top of the right column.

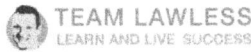

TEAM LAWLESS
LEARN AND LIVE SUCCESS

Going-Away Things

Everything that causes me depression, boredom, being overwhelmed, anger, worry, frustration, resentment, sadness, jealousy, self-pity

Going-Away Things	Limiting Beliefs
My weight	I cannot live without bread, pasta, and wine.
Hypos at night	I need a few glasses of wine at night to calm me down.

Then head to the next chapter, where you will narrow your focus to the few beliefs that you can change to make the most positive impact on the quality of your diabetes life.

CHAPTER FIVE

Step 2: Create Your Wheel of Diabetes Mastery™

Congratulations on making it through Step 1. This is huge. You got it all out. How do you feel? A good sign is if the weight on your shoulders is a bit lighter, but you are also a little scared. This typically means that you are stimulated for growth and ready to commit to progress.

Deep down in your heart, you know that bottling it all up will make it worse. What would it mean to you if you held onto your limiting beliefs? How would your life be 5, 10, or 20 years from now if you didn't change? What legacy will you leave behind when you die? What will your children say about you in your eulogy?

My own biggest nightmare is that when I die, I will meet the person I could have become in life. That's why I have a framed quote from the designer and sculptor of the Crazy Horse Memorial, Korczak Ziolkowski, in my office:

The world asks you one question, only one: "Did you do the job?" And there is only one answer: "Yes." You don't say, "I would have done it if there had been any money in it." You don't say, "I would have done it if people had been more sympathetic and understood what I was trying to do." You don't say, "I would have done it if I hadn't gotten hurt or crippled"—and, God knows, I've been crippled. You don't even say, "I would have done the job if I hadn't died." I don't buy that. There is only one answer: "Yes."

Let's get real and paint a picture of where you stand and then work toward your yes. You will not need the results from your latest blood work, A1c trend lines, or food inventory. Instead, I will guide you through the process with a few questions. You will then rate your current situation based on how you feel. When you give your answers, don't paint your picture better or worse than it is. Be honest with yourself and remember that the one person you are hardest on is yourself.

A good way of illustrating your current starting point is to do a Wheel of Diabetes Mastery™ exercise.

Download the full worksheet in my Facebook group or from the resource page for this book which you can find at http://BloodSugarInCheck.com.

Wheel of Diabetes Mastery Worksheet

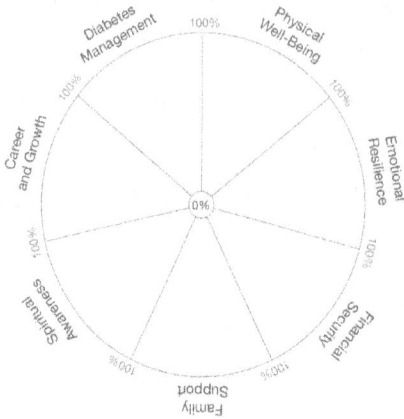

My Focus Area is: _____

What is already good about my Focus Area
1. _____
2. _____
3. _____

What I have learned about my Focus Area:
1. _____
2. _____
3. _____

What I am willing to do to make it how I want it:
1. _____
2. _____
3. _____

What I am willing to not do to make it how I want it:
1. _____
2. _____
3. _____

There are seven pie pieces in the Wheel of Diabetes Mastery™, with each representing a vital area of management. Think through each area in your wheel and draw a horizontal line across every pie piece at a level between 0 and 100. Zero means that you have nothing; 100 says that you have everything. Don't overthink your ratings. Go with your gut. That's why there are no numbers on the scale between 0% and 100% Just put the line where it feels right. You can—and will make adjustments later on. Whether you believe you are at 30%, 50%, or 70% in any given category, just draw a line from left to right in the pie piece with the corresponding label.

At the end of this exercise, your Wheel of Diabetes Mastery™ should look like the example below, only your lines will be at different values in each pie piece.

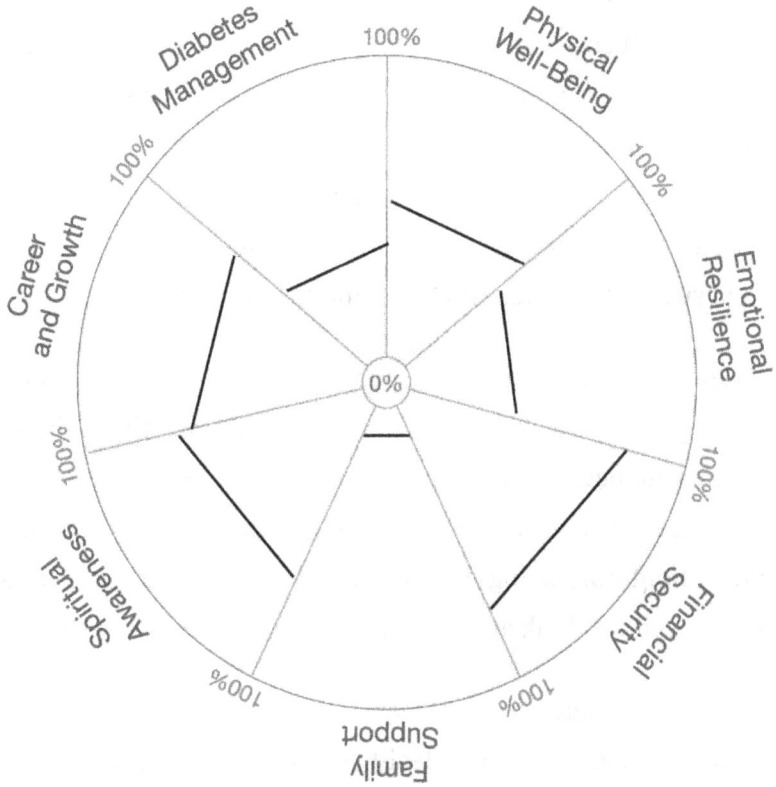

Wheel of Diabetes Mastery™ Questions

Diabetes Management

How well do you control your blood sugar? If you are on a perpetual glucose roller coaster, then your line should probably be closer to 0. If you are relatively stable and your A1c is below 7, then you are closer to 100%. How often do you measure your blood sugar? If you prick your fingers 5 to 7 times a day and keep a journal, then you are closer to 100%. If you never measure your blood sugar at all, then draw the line closer to 0%.

Remember that this is a judgment-free zone. No one is perfect. We have all failed ourselves multiple times in our diabetes management. Being honest with yourself is the first step. Draw the line where you feel it belongs, without judgment and without portraying it as worse or better than it really is. No one but you will look at your results, unless you want to share it.

If your diabetes management really sucks right now, then capture it exactly how you feel based on what you know, what you do, and what you do not do. With these thoughts in mind, ask yourself the following additional questions about your diabetes management.

How is your diet? Are you feasting on pizza and ice cream, or do you adhere to an alkaline diet? These are two extremes, and most of us zigzag between them. Most people do not eat pizza all the time, and only a few will deny themselves all eating pleasures. Don't worry if you do live in extremes. What you need to determine is how healthy you believe your diet is overall. There is no judgment anywhere in this book or in my mind. Neither should it be in your head.

How regularly and effectively do you take your medication to keep your blood sugar in check? If you have stopped taking pills or insulin altogether, then move your line closer to 0%. If you have this part of diabetes management under control, then elevate it toward 100%.

Physical Well-Being

Do you make healthy lifestyle choices that support your diabetes management? Do you get enough sleep? Are you building muscular and cardiovascular strength? Do you have an established exercise routine? Do you eat healthily? Move your lines up if you can answer yes. Do you smoke and consume large amounts of alcohol, sugar, caffeine, or empty calories? Bring the line down.

Other factors that move the line are: How intimately are you engaged in developing your physical wellness? Do you know your critical health numbers, such as cholesterol, weight, blood pressure, and blood sugar levels? Do you feel energized?

If you haven't worked out in the past 6 months, live on fast food, smoke, drink alcohol, and are overweight, then your line will be closer to 0. If healthy choices are a part of your daily routine, and you feel energetic with an active lifestyle, then you are closer to 100.

Don't overthink it. I know a supertoned fitness trainer and yoga teacher who feels she is at 50% of her physical well-being. Meanwhile, I thought I was at 60%, even though I had had type 1 diabetes for more than 40 years and was less toned and slightly overweight when I spoke to her. How you feel is based on what you know, what you do, and what you do not do. Here, I want you to determine how healthy you believe your diet is overall. Again, no judgment.

Do you drink an ounce of water for each pound you weigh, every day? Great. Your line in the pie just went up a notch. Do you drink less, or do you live on diet soda and coffee? Move the line down.

Emotional Resilience

How do you handle stress? Does your blood sugar easily skyrocket under stress? If yes, then move the line close to 0%. Are you able to live and work independently while seeking and appreciating the support and friendship of others? Bring the line up.

How well are you aware of your thoughts and feelings about your diabetes? Do you feel that it is unfair that you cannot eat the foods you love, cannot live as freely as you would like, or have to worry about your blood sugar levels all the time? Do you often wonder, *Why me?* and feel self-pity? Are you afraid that people will judge you for having diabetes and, as a result, you do not take your medication at work or at a party? Move the line down.

If your outlook on life is positive despite your illness, and you accept and love yourself with diabetes, then move the line up. If you feel depressed or sad most of the time, then bring it down.

How would you rate your social life and the depth of your friendships? Do you enjoy the time you spend with others?

Take all your answers into consideration and draw a line.

Financial Security

Can you afford your illness? People with diabetes have health care costs 2.3 times greater than those without diabetes. How well can you absorb these extra costs? Or do you struggle to maintain costs? That happens to 45% of diabetics in the US. If you feel the financial impact of diabetes, then move the line closer to 0%. If you are among the lucky ones who can pay for the additional cost and then some, then your line will be closer to 100%.

How much control do you have over your day-to-day and month-to-month finances as a result of your diabetes? Do you hardly feel the impact, or are you struggling to make ends meet? What do you give up as a result? Are you on track to achieve your financial goals? How much are you saving to generate compound interest to grow your wealth and ensure retirement?

Family Support

Do you have fun together as a family and build strong, loving bonds? Or are you thinking that you have done this diabetes thing to yourself and so here you are, alone? Are you afraid that you could face amputation, or any major surgery, alone?

Then draw a line close to 0%.

If, on the other hand, your family is working with you as a unit to manage your diabetes health, then bring the line further up. How well you manage your diabetes is directly dependent on the amount of support you receive from your family. Do they listen to what you think and feel? Do you listen to them? Do they support or even join you in making healthy changes, such as everyone adopting an alkaline diet or becoming your running buddies? Do they have realistic expectations about your blood glucose levels and avoid blame?

Do you feel valued for making a contribution and taking on responsibilities? Do you have enough quality time to relax or spend meaningful moments with your family? Or are you preoccupied with your illness? How often and how many meals do you eat together? What is the quality of your dinner conversations? How much time do you take to listen to and show interest in your family members? Who loves you? What about you do they love? How does it feel to be loved by them? These answers may be hardest to measure. They are also the most emotional.

This is the one pie piece in the Wheel of Diabetes Mastery™ that makes you cry the most when you think through the answers to the questions. Letting your tears flow begins the healing. Acknowledge the hurt inside and then let it go. Remember that every emotion is a call to action.

Hurt, for example, is a signal that you have an expectation that is not being met, and you may need to change your way of communicating your needs or change your behavior. Anger means that an important rule that you have in your life has been violated, and you may need to clarify your rules or adjust them. Guilt is a signal that you broke one of your own standards and may need to make things right. Feeling unworthy is a signal that you need to do something better. Loneliness is a signal that you need a connection with people, and you may need to find a better peer group.

Very often, the only thing we can do is love our families but choose our peers. Just draw a line for now where you feel things are. You will take action in Step 4.

Spiritual Awareness

Spiritual awareness does not necessarily mean affiliation with a religion. It does not even suggest that you need to have a belief in a higher authority at all. Although you might. I am not here to tell anyone what they need to believe. We all get our spirituality from different sources.

Spiritually means that you have a clear sense of direction and purpose for your life and that you accept yourself with diabetes. It says that you are allowing yourself to be present in the here and now and not letting your mind continually worry over long-term complications or potential hypoglycemia attacks (hypos). It means that you have a keen appreciation of the wonders of nature and its possibilities and feel grateful for your blessings, possessions, and friendships. Draw a line closer to 100% if you feel that way. Bring it down if you don't.

How well are you connected with your inner being? Do you meditate, pray, or practice mindfulness? Do you experience a higher intrinsic meaning in life and inner peace? Adjust your line according to your answer.

Career and Growth

Let's be honest. People with diabetes take 2 more sick days per year than healthy people. Productivity losses from diabetes in American companies add up to about $40 billion per year. Several studies find negative associations between diabetics and business outcomes. How do these data points impact you?

Do you face discrimination, for example, because you do not have access to jobs that are safety sensitive because of your risk of hypoglycemia? Office workers can usually manage their diabetes without it affecting their work, but some, for example, do not take on shift work because it messes with the timing of their medication and diet. If you experience such limited job choices, then move the line closer to 0.

If you have access to regular meal breaks, can step out of a meeting quickly to get your blood sugar back up, and have the ability to test your blood sugar level, then your line can move closer to 100.

Are you doing what you are meant to do? Or does your diabetes keep you from matching your talents to the needs of the world? Do you feel you can or cannot pursue your dream job?

Are you able to use your strengths, or do you work against your grain most of the time? Do you receive meaningful recognition for your contributions? How do you rate the relationship between you and your manager? Do you have your supervisor's support to take care of your diabetes at work? Are you professionally growing? Do you have a least one true friend at work who looks out for you in case you need help during a hypo?

If you can honestly say, "I am cool. My vocation is my calling. I am fulfilled, energized, and fully motivated," then you can put the line at 100%. If you are continually holding back, wanting to punch your coworkers, clients, and manager in the face, then you are at 0.

Just draw a line where you think things are going for you today.

How Fast Can You Go and How Smoothly?

Scribble your pie pieces solid and then ask yourself, if this Wheel of Diabetes Mastery™ were the four wheels on your car, how fast could you go? How smooth would the ride be?

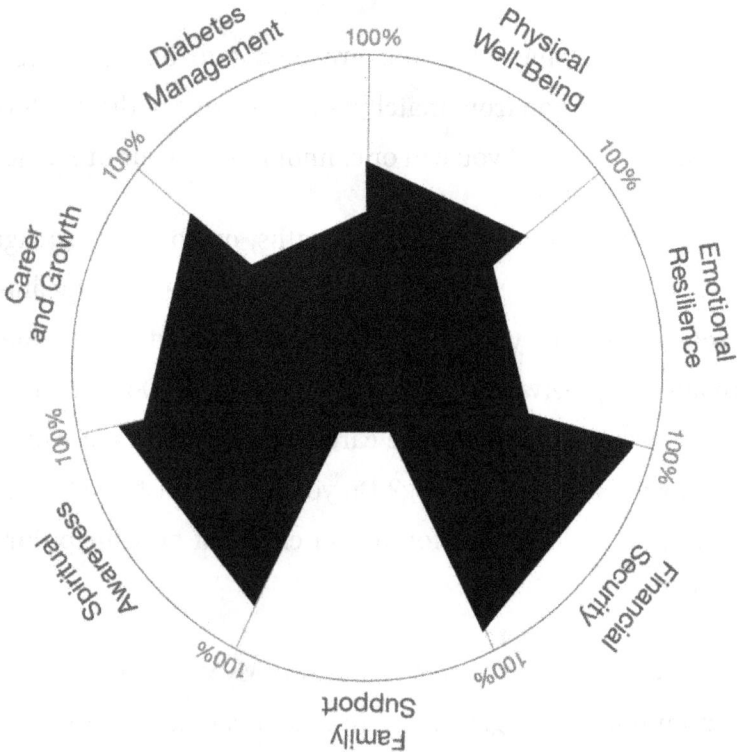

If you are like most people, then your Wheel of Diabetes Mastery™ will look rough, with some pie pieces stronger than others. Everyone's wheel does at this juncture. That's why in my workshops, I ask participants to share their Wheel of Diabetes Mastery™ with the rest of the group, so they see that everyone created that same slow, bumpy ride.

Let's Smooth Out Your Wheel

I am so proud of you. I know the feeling when you first look at your Wheel of Diabetes Mastery™ and scream inside your head, *I am screwed! I am not good enough to make this go away.*

Stop that voice inside your head right now. Remember that acknowledging and owning your situation is the first step to improvement. You are one step closer to a better future with diabetes.

Look at it this way: Success is a result of sound judgment, which, in turn, comes from experience, which is often a result of mistakes that you made in the past. Mistakes, finally, are a matter of bad judgment. Your Wheel of Diabetes Mastery™ reflects mistakes or specific actions that you took in the past. So what? With every mistake, you gained experience and got one step closer to better health and happiness with diabetes. You would not have bought this book if you had not made mistakes in the past and continued to make mistakes now.

You will be using these experiences now to make your life with diabetes the way you want it and get the results that you deserve.

What Are You the Master of?

Look at your Wheel of Diabetes Mastery™. There is most likely one area that you are good at—or at least better at than others. An area that you have mastered to some degree. Which area is that?

At this point, you may feel like you must improve every area of life with diabetes. In your mind, all may need work, and that can be overwhelming. Do not despair. You will make it manageable shortly.

You may be the master of your physical well-being or your financial security. Some people are emotionally strong, even though the world around them collapses. Others build their strongest family bonds in times of financial adversity. I am sure that you, too, have one area you do better in than others. What is the one area you are good at? What is something over which you have the most control? Identify which one that is and put a star on the corresponding pie piece.

The next area of management you need to identify is the one that would impact all others if you built it out. For example, you could say, "If I felt better physically, I could do my job better. That, in turn, would have an impact on my finances, and I would have the time to take care of my diabetes." But this may not be true for everybody.

Another person with diabetes may say, "You know what? If I had more support from my family and I felt better emotionally, it would give me the mental energy to do better and manage my blood sugar well. Then I could worry about everything else, or otherwise, I won't function."

There is no right or wrong answer. Every life, every person, is unique. Another person with diabetes could have created a similar Wheel of Diabetes Mastery™ and concluded, "If only I had a more inspiring boss, I would be less stressed at home and could focus on my kids instead of worrying about my work. So, let me find a new job first, and then I will make a positive impact on at least two or three other areas."

You may not have the best answer for yourself right now, but I want you to keep finding the one area that you can improve, rather than improving everything at once. If you try to change everything, guess what will happen. Nothing. You are attempting to boil the ocean. This may be the number one reason most plans fail: They are too complex. When I worked at The World Bank, I always chuckled when I heard the term "comprehensive plan." To this day I interpret it as a preemptive excuse for not achieving results.

That's why I want you to pick a single area of impact. Which one will positively affect everything else? Think that through right now, because you will continue to work within that focus area for the remainder of this book. Stop reading for a moment and reflect.

A question I often get at this stage is whether the Wheel of Diabetes Mastery™ needs to be built out on the personal level or for the entire team/family. Right now, it's all about you. We will get to the people in your life another time, in another book or in my coaching sessions, if you want to join them. For now, understand that the Wheel of Diabetes Mastery™ will change over time. Half a year from now, you will draw a new wheel, because you will have made progress and can move on.

Remember that you are not your past until you die. You can move your life in a different direction in an instant and at every moment. If you have ever made a decision that changed your life completely, for better or worse, then you know what I am talking about. When was the last time you made such a decision? You can make it at any time.

Five Answers to Get You on a Healthy Path

Now that you know the one area that you need to build out to improve your overall relationship with diabetes, ask yourself five questions that will help you find your own solutions for living a happy and healthy life with diabetes.

1. What is your question?

Frame your situation into a quality question. Stating that your situation sucks, allowing self-pity, or telling yourself that you are not good enough will not help you find a solution.

When my 7-year-old son, Dylan, complains about anything, my response is usually, "What's your question?" Every complaint is a question not asked or a cry for help. When he complains, "There is no food in the fridge," he actually means he does not like the food he sees and wants to eat something other than what's on display.

The voice inside your head is like my 7-year-old son when he opens the fridge. It first sees and focuses on the negative. It does not automatically see solutions. You will need to make the nagging stop and replace it with empowering questions.

Whenever you find yourself in a tricky situation, and especially when you feel anxious, depressed, or angry about your diabetes in general or your blood sugar roller coaster, step back and ask yourself, *What's the question?*

In the beginning, my son would respond with yet another complaint: "I don't like the food in the fridge." So, I would respond, "I hear you. What can I do to make you feel better? What's your question?" The mind does not always switch easily unless it has been trained to do so. In the beginning, it takes a lot of reinforcement and repetition.

Eventually, Dylan would say, "I don't like salad. Can we make something else?" That statement is already better. It's actionable. So I would offer him a vegan sausage, knowing that he does not like it either, because I wanted him to phrase a solution-oriented question.

The quality of a question matters. It has to be specific, measurable, actionable, realistic, and time driven (SMART goals). Eventually, Dylan learned to ask the question as follows: "How can we make a yummy dinner with the ingredients that we have in the fridge and pantry before Mummy comes home?" A yummy dinner may not be specific enough you, but for Dylan, it means it needs to include chocolate (think Nutella), cucumbers, chickpeas, shrimp, pasta, cheese, or pizza. So, for him, it is a smart question.

Ask better questions, get better answers. Every emotion, every complaint, is a question that wants to be uncovered. As Dylan puts it today, "Think solutions, not problems." I love hearing that from a 7-year-old as much as I like hearing it from grown-ups. It never gets old.

2. What's great about your diabetes?

Asking a quality question is designed to quiet that self-doubting voice of yours and get your mind into a solution-finding mode. The purpose of the second question is to keep you there and strengthen your mindset.

Have you ever sat at your desk, scratching your head, pressing your fingers into the creases of your forehead, and trying to find a solution for a significant problem? In that state, have you actually ever come up with the best answers? If your response is no, then you are not alone. You cannot be creative in a tense mental state.

Compare that with times when you are in a great mood. People who are in love, for example, believe they can do anything they put their minds to. And often they can, while people under severe stress merely perform.

Ask yourself what is good about diabetes or your specific struggle with the disease. It keeps your brain away from doing what it is designed to do best: figure out a way to survive. But you do not want to merely endure; you want to succeed and live your diabetes life in better health and with more happiness.

You can always, always find something that is good about even the darkest moment. "Rock bottom became the solid foundation on which I rebuilt my life," writes *Harry Potter* author and billionaire J. K. Rowling. When she was as poor as it is possible to be in Britain without being homeless, she was "set free," she says, "because my greatest fear had been realized, and I was still alive, and I still had a daughter whom I adored. And I had an old typewriter and a big idea."

For the area in your Wheel of Diabetes Mastery™ that you want to build out first, find at least three things that are great. I know that often it feels like there is nothing good. Then think about what could be good if you wanted it to be. Can you walk, talk, and use your mind? You are already better off than many other people. Australian Nick Vujicic was born with no arms or legs, yet he wrote a book, *Life Without Limits: Inspiration for a Ridiculously Good Life,* which has been translated into over 30 languages. He has moved, coached, and changed people in more than 57 countries on topics such as bullying, inspiring positive change, persistence, determination, and his own life story. His core message: "No matter your circumstance, you can overcome!" Would he have inspired so many people if he had been born without complications?

Diabetes keeps you busy, and it can be annoying. It also helps you build critical character traits. Diabetes is the reason I have always been more resilient than most people in my life and have taken on more responsibilities than others. I wrote my first best-selling book when I was 23 years old, interviewed Bill Gates exclusively for *Forbes* magazine in Germany at 25, and worked as an editor in chief at 26. All because diabetes instilled discipline in me that others did not need at that age.

What's good about your life with diabetes?

3. What can you learn?

This is another question that keeps your mind focused on the solution. Remember that success is a matter of experience, which, in turn, is the result of having made mistakes. By asking yourself what you can learn, you harness the power of mistakes and turn them into valuable experiences that eventually lead to better health and more happiness with diabetes. You will make sure that you do not make the same mistakes again and instead find new ways to approach life.

Find at least three lessons from your current situation that can help you achieve better health, sanity, and happiness with diabetes. Maybe you have learned that potatoes spike your blood sugar more than any other food or that eating pizza requires much more thought than just injecting the usual amount of insulin per carbohydrate. Maybe you have learned that your family will be there for you and know what to do when you are about to pass out from a hypo. Or the opposite may be true: You have learned that you need to educate them better and have alternative strategies in place.

There is always something to learn.

4. What's not perfect about your diabetes yet?

This question is different from, "What is not great?" or "What is not working?" which focus on the problem. Asking yourself what's not perfect yet presupposes a desirable outcome. It implies that your situation will be perfect eventually.

Nonetheless, you will need to persistently focus your mind on finding a solution, instead of dwelling on the problem. Your brain is naturally wired to see what can harm you. It makes it easy for you to give negative answers. Your job is to rephrase those answers in vision-oriented ways.

Do not say, "I do not have enough money." Instead, say something like, "I need five more paying clients" or "I need a better-paying job." You can also say, "I do not need any money to start living healthily tomorrow. All I need to do to is put on my running shoes and run."

You may not be able to state a problem in a mission-driven way all the time, but at least try.

One of the most impactful responsibilities in my job as a coach is to keep my clients in a positive mindset while they are working through these initial questions. I find them too often drifting back into the negative. They say something like: "I need a better job, but I do not have enough qualifications." When that happens, I ask my clients to replace the word "but" with "and": "I need a better job and I do not have enough qualifications" already sounds better. The brain works differently. Replacing the word "but" with the word "and" makes it easier to turn the second part of the sentence into an action-oriented statement, such as, "I need a better job and one that needs my talents."

Your brain will not give up trying to pull you into survival mode. Your mind will have to pull back constantly. Language matters. What you say to yourself is essential. So are the questions you ask yourself. "How can I get my message across?" is a better question than "Why does no one understand me?"

5. What am I willing to do to make it how I want it?

This question also looks forward. Some people with diabetes ask themselves questions like, "How do I make diabetes go away?" They are dwelling on the problem, even though they know there is no cure for the disease, whether it is type 1 or type 2 diabetes.

"What caused my diabetes?"

"Were my eating habits responsible?"

"Why are health insurance co-pays so high?"

"Why me?"

On Facebook, I see two types of people: those who are consumed by the pains of diabetes and those who look forward to the wonders and opportunities in their lives. The ones with a positive outlook focus no more than 20% of their energy on the problem and 80% on the solution. The miserable do the opposite.

Coming-in Things

Keep it positive and fire along. Here is a chance to build your massive action plan. Now is the time to keep your ideas flowing on your "Coming-In Things" worksheet. You can find it in my

Facebook group [4]files or download it from the resource website for this book at http://BloodSugarInCheck.com.

List in the left column all the things you want to come into your life. Coming-in things include everything that brings you happiness, love, health, success, intelligence, power, growth, contribution, affection, and humor.

Only write in the left column and leave the right one empty for now. As with your Going-Away Things list, continue on a second copy of this worksheet if you run out of space.

Make sure no one disturbs you and nothing distracts you during this exercise. Turn off everything that can get divert your attention while you write. Turn off your notifications on your laptop, phone, tablet, smart watch, smart speakers, and anything else that can give you an alert. You are about to discover new insights and strategies. You deserve this time.

Do not continue reading this book until you have completed this exercise. The rest of this book relies on the outcome of the alignment of your behavioral forces. You will benefit from reading the following chapters without completing your list of coming-in things, but you will only be able to take full advantage of all strategies once you have written your thoughts down.

Start writing now.

---

[4] Facebook Page *https://www.facebook.com/groups/diabetesmentor*

When you are done, your list may now look like this:

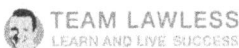

TEAM LAWLESS
LEARN AND LIVE SUCCESS

Coming-In Things

Everything that brings me happiness, love, health, success, intelligence, power,
growth, contribution, affection, humor

Coming-In Things

Alc 6.5	
Encouragement and praise from my family	
More fun	
Better health care	
More and better sex	
Eating out more often	
Practicing yoga	

Align Your Two Behavioral Forces

Now cross-reference your list of coming-in things with your list of going-away things, and cross off everything that you cannot find on both lists. For example, if one of your going-away things is "low sex drive," then you will need to find a corresponding entry on the list of coming-in things, such as "more and better sex" or "more intimacy."

Your matching list could look like this:

Going-Away Things	Coming-In Things
My weight	Having lost weight
Extreme high blood sugar	A1c 6.5
Worry over long-term complications	A1c 6.5
Restrictive diet	More exciting food
Daily stress of managing my diabetes	Encouragement and praise from my family
Low sex drive	More and better sex

As you can see from the example above, two items on the first list of coming-in things are no longer on the second list of coming-in things: better health care and practicing yoga. This does not mean that these items are no longer important for the fictional person who put together both lists. They are just not his or her highest priority right now. If they were, then they would have been mentioned on both lists.

Here is where the two forces that drive your behavior come together. The reason items are on both lists is because of your need to avoid pain. For example, "restrictive diet" is aligned with your desire to gain pleasure, i.e. "eating out more often."

You have now created further clarity in your mind about what you need to do and narrowed down your strategy to a smaller number of outcomes that will give you results. Your brain and your mind know what you need. And now so do you.

Turn Your Diabetes Grief into Empowering Beliefs

Help your mind make sure your brain stays on track. Remember that your brain actively sabotages you when you want to make drastic changes. You will, therefore, now borrow from Alicia Crum's recipe and begin to mind-wrestle your autonomous nervous system into success.

If you remember, in her experiments, Crum stopped people from being hungry just by showing them a nutrition label that made them believe that they had consumed a tremendous number of calories, even if they had not. She managed to help cleaning personnel lower their blood pressure by giving them a 15-minute PowerPoint presentation on how their job meets the criteria for a healthy lifestyle.

You will now create your own presentation and labels.

One of the reasons people with diabetes, for example, feel their families are not supportive is often because they make negative associations. A voice inside their head tells them that they brought the disease on themselves, and that they are too ugly, fat, or unworthy to be loved. If you think of yourself in these terms, then it is hard to imagine that someone else loves you and cares for you.

If you want your family's support, then begin with changing your own focus from your habitual feelings of low self-worth to a new belief. One trick for loving and valuing yourself more is to follow a process called neuro-associative conditioning (NAC). You must change how you associate your situation with your feelings and beliefs; otherwise, your old forces will pull you back into old territory in no time.

You will learn more about NAC in Step 5 of your Diabetes Mastery™ process. In this step, you'll begin by radically changing what you say to yourself. You will turn your limiting beliefs from Step 1 into empowering statements.

Instead of saying, "I cannot live without bread, pasta, and potatoes," you could say, "Trying and experimenting with new foods together is a great way of reconnecting with my husband." Instead of saying, "I will never be good at managing my diabetes," you could say, "I decide how I live my life, not diabetes. I manage it and live my life. I am not a victim, no matter what happens!"

Link pleasure to your new choice and say it to yourself as often as you can. Give yourself the speech, the presentation, or that new label all the time. Repetition is vital, because your brain does not differentiate between story and reality. The more often you make these new associations, the more likely they will become your new life.

You will begin that process in the next step, where you will decide on the specific action to achieve your goals. You will determine which activities keep you in the flow and motivated to keep on setting new standards and stepping up.

CHAPTER SIX

Step 3: Design Your Personal Diabetes Plan

Wow! You now have a list of meaningful goals for your Diabetes Mastery™, and you have created statements for yourself that empower you to take action. You have also discovered that you must mind-wrestle your brain into success.

In Step 3, we will take a closer look at your mind and then begin beating it into submission.

We tend to talk about the mind as one entity, but it has three parts, or layers, that need to work in the same direction for you to succeed or fail:

1. The first is the cognitive layer, which houses what we know, our skills, and experience.

2. The second, the affective layer, determines how you relate to other people, your value system, what drives you, and your motivation.

3. The third layer is called the conative, which holds the key to how you initiate action. This layer is at the core of this step in your diabetes transformation process, because it is responsible for what you will and will not do to manage your diabetes.

Here is how the three parts work.

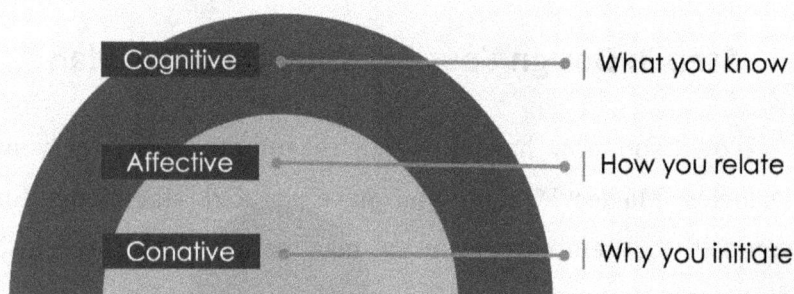

Cognitive	What you know
Affective	How you relate
Conative	Why you initiate

© 2012 – 2018 Andrew Lawless & Rockant, Inc.

Do You Know Enough About Diabetes Management?

The gray matter of your brain, the neocortex, holds all your knowledge, experiences, and judgment. That is where the cognitive layer of the mind sits. Here is where you solve math problems, translate documents, or remember facts. It is also the part of both the brain and the mind where language resides.

When you walk into a store to buy a television and find yourself comparing features and technical specifications, that's when the cognitive part of your mind is reeling. You know how it can mess with you if you have ever gone back and forth between two TVs or laptop models and found it hard to make a decision. And if you did make a decision, took your choice home, and then wondered if you should have bought the other one, then congratulations: You have experienced the power of confusion of the cognitive mind.

You probably experienced the same level of uncertainty in managing your diabetes when you were first diagnosed. At that time, you knew as much about diabetes as most people understand about a computer's RAM, GB, and MHz. You just did not have enough knowledge, experience, or judgment yet to medicate yourself, count carbohydrates, understand the effect of alcohol on your blood sugar levels, and so on.

That's an easy fix: Your diabetes care team is most likely well equipped to teach you all you need to know. There are also plenty of free and paid resources you can access by Googling whatever you want to know. You do not even have to read anymore. Your YouTube app on your tablet gives you the ability to use voice search to find video instructions.

You must love technology. Use it to stay in active communication with your diabetes care team about what you do or plan to change.

Do Your Habits Still Serve You with Diabetes?

Have you ever wanted to drive to the gym or church on a Sunday morning and ended up in front of your office instead? That's the affective layer of your mind working. This part of the mind houses your values, beliefs, and motivations. It also holds the behavioral patterns that put you on autopilot.

The affective layer is conditioned based on many social factors. Early in life, your parents encouraged specific behaviors and reinforced their values. Your friends, teachers, work environment, colleagues, and life experience shaped the affective part of your mind throughout the rest of your life. For example, just ask anyone who likes coffee, whiskey, wine, nicotine, or olives if they loved it the first time they tried it. Most of them will say, "No. I hated it. It was bad" or, "The first time that I smoked, I felt like I needed to throw up."

Why, then, have they continued to smoke or drink coffee or whiskey and continue to do this to their bodies? The answer is that they have conditioned themselves to like it by succumbing to the two forces that shape behavior in all of us. We covered them in Step 1 in your Diabetes Mastery™ process: the need to avoid pain and the desire to gain pleasure.

Smoking is a good example. People who smoke often report that they just wanted to fit in with their peer group, in which everyone smoked. Not smoking would have made them the oddball, and the pain of being isolated, laughed at, ignored, or not respected was more significant than the pain of inhaling cigarette smoke. At the same time, they wanted to have all the fun that comes with being a member of this peer group and maybe even enjoyed the experience of being cool, with a cigarette in their hands. In other words, they conditioned themselves to like smoking because of all the pleasure that they perceived it would give them—and eventually began craving the nicotine.

The problem with cigarettes is that they may have served smokers in these ways in the past, but they do more harm than good in the long term. To quit cigarettes, smokers must recondition themselves as hard as they did when they were determined to like cigarettes. They can use all kinds of tools, from nicotine patches to hypnotherapy, and it usually takes at least 3 weeks to stabilize new routines and behavioral patterns. To stay away from cigarettes, they will need at least another 9 weeks to make it stick.

Which is why my Diabetes Mastery™ program spans 12 weeks, with an option for ongoing support after that. By the way, if you want to know more about Diabetes Mastery™ coaching, check out the resource page for this book on the web at http://bloodsugarincheck.com or send me an email to andrew@bloodsugarincheck.com.

The concept of changing behavioral patterns is similar to that of tuning a piano. No piano will stay in tune forever. Hot, cold, and wet weather move and swell its parts, which are made from wood, metal, felt, and leather. Over time, these environmental forces change the pitch and tone of each key. When a piano has not been tuned for a while, a professional tuning expert will come in and fix it. They start tuning the first key and work themselves all the way up the keyboard to the highest one.

Then something interesting happens. If the piano has not been looked after for a long time, the lowest key will already be out of tune the moment the tuning professional has completed work on the highest one. The old forces continue to pull in old directions. The piano will need to be tuned once every week initially, then once a month, and once a quarter until it becomes a twice yearly or annual routine.

You'll change the way you feel about your diabetes the same way. In the beginning, you will need to retune the affective layer of your mind in smaller intervals before you can go into maintenance mode. In Step 5 of your Diabetes Mastery™ process, you will dig deeper into the mechanics of how to recondition yourself.

For now, understand that the affective layer of the mind negatively impacts your blood sugar levels. The most obvious reasons are the routines that you followed before your diagnosis are no longer serving you, and you need to replace them with new ones. It often starts with just a small decision, such as waking up earlier in the morning than usual and taking a brisk, 30-minute walk around the block instead of starting your day with pancakes and coffee.

Do You Work Against the Grain in Your Diabetes Care?

When it comes to managing diabetes, some people seem to be naturally wired to plan their meals for the week ahead, how many carbohydrates they will eat for each meal, and how much medication they will take. They do not even need much training. They are intuitive planners. These are the people who check the restaurant menu ahead of time and know in advance what they will eat and when and how much medication to take.

Other people with diabetes deal with whatever comes up. They check what is on their plate when it is being served and make decisions at that very moment. They don't think through which restaurant they will go to and instead figure out meal orders and their dosage of medication as things come up. This may even include, for example, injecting more insulin during dinner when they realize that they will eat much more food than they had anticipated. They are naturally born shortcutters.

While we all follow some version of these two approaches, we cannot have the instincts for both. Especially when under stress or time pressure, we revert to what the conative part of the mind wants us to do. Shortcutters will easily ignore protocols for best practices in blood sugar control that systematizers have created for them. Or they will try hard without getting positive results – then burnout. The following diagram illustrates how you can fail to manage your diabetes on the three levels of the mind. Right now, we are focusing on the conative part.

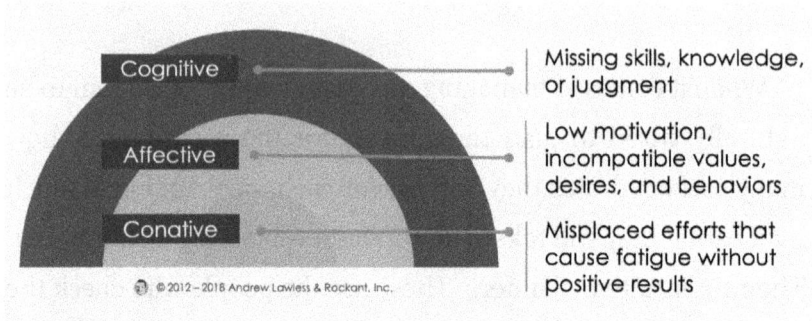

Cognitive	Missing skills, knowledge, or judgment
Affective	Low motivation, incompatible values, desires, and behaviors
Conative	Misplaced efforts that cause fatigue without positive results

© 2012 – 2018 Andrew Lawless & Rockant, Inc.

This level of the mind drives the way we take action. I have seen in my own experience how my instinctive strengths sometimes undermine the advice from doctors, nutritionists, and diabetes educators.

I am willing to take more risks with my diabetes management than others. When going into town, I rarely have sugar tablets or jelly beans on me that I can eat when my blood sugar drops too low, for example. I figure there is always a shop nearby when I need it. I am also convinced that having jelly beans on me already sets an expectation in my mind that I will have a hypo, whereas not having them in my pocket prepares my mind for keeping my blood sugar steadier. This may sound crazy to you, and if it does, it most likely won't work for you. But it serves me most of the time; when it doesn't, there is a shop right around the corner, where I can buy juice. At other times, my wife has my back with a candy bar in her purse.

The art of Diabetes Mastery™ is to make diabetes management work for you, not the other way around. You are most likely different from me, so do not follow my practices. Instead, collaborate closely with your diabetes care team and remember to include your significant other, family, friends, and colleagues.

My wife, for example, is my opposite. While I like to rock the boat, she naturally stabilizes. She minimizes risk and plans ahead. Hence, she keeps a candy bar in her purse in case I need it. She is also the one who reminds me to bring my insulin pen and glucose meter. Most of the time she even knows where I left them when I cannot find them. There is an excellent synergy between us, and her talents are a great rock for me to stand on.

This did not happen by accident. We had to make it work. In fact, Ann's robotic nature used to annoy me, and on the flip side, she felt that I often made communication about my medical needs difficult because I gave too many options. Ann is sharp like a knife and steady like a train. I learn by challenging boundaries and experimenting; I sprint and change my mind quickly.

Have you ever noticed that some people with diabetes neatly file their latest blood work results, while others cannot remember the last time they took their A1c or what it was? This level of organization is deeply ingrained in their minds, and this deep programming makes it hard for some to use apps and journals, while others do this naturally.

There is no right or wrong way. For example, I have always relied on shortcuts and used technology as much to my advantage as possible to keep track of and chart my blood sugar levels over time rather than forcing myself to use a process that I tend not to follow for long.

I have seen friends who did not use their natural strengths in their health care and developed diabetes burnout as a result. It affects 44% of people diagnosed with either type 1 or type 2 diabetes. It happens at any age, and a variety of events can trigger it: high A1c over a long time, trouble in a relationship, family issues, the death of a loved one, or the first sign of complications.

But diabetes burnout does not pop up overnight. Yes, a divorce or breakup, a death in the family, or a medical diagnosis can and will throw all of us off. But these traumatic events do not necessarily lead to giving up on diabetes care. Most likely, people with diabetes burnout did not get enough positive results from their blood sugar management and feel depressed by the lack of success. They were working against their grain all the time, and then at one point, a small trigger event broke their willpower altogether.

In Step 5 of your Diabetes Mastery™ process, you will dig deeper into the mechanics of how to recondition yourself. For now, let's look at the bigger picture.

Use Your Diabetes Instincts

Believe it or not, how you start a new diet, measure and track your blood sugar levels and carbs, plan your shopping trips, and even find and put together your diabetes care team are pretty much always the same. You have acquired these behavioral and problem-solving patterns throughout your life.

My wife, Ann, for example, always creates a plan of attack before she does anything. She goes shopping with a list of healthy food items based on what we want to cook. My school of grocery shopping is different. I will suddenly decide that I need to buy more almond milk and drive to the supermarket ad hoc. Once in the shopping aisles, I will put into the cart whatever else I see that excites me. "Hey, there is a new fancy box of oat milk available? Let's get that, even if we have just stocked up with a different brand. And how about the coconut yogurt? Have not had that in a while." Into the cart it goes. I do not remember ever using a shopping list, apart from the ones that Ann texts me when she knows that I am on the way to the store.

How we conduct research about the qualifications of our doctors and keep a list that journals our blood sugar levels, carbohydrates, and medication intake are most likely also always the same or at least similar. The reason I forget to bring jelly beans with me is that I organize on the fly. I do not plan and think ahead that much, which serves me most of the time but can also get me into great trouble.

One time, I was on a flight to China that was so turbulent, flight attendants strapped themselves to their chairs and would not speak or get up, even when one of their service carts went tumbling. When that happens, you know it is serious. There was no food or service for about an hour, and I suddenly realized that I urgently needed to eat, because my blood sugar had dropped. As a risk-taker and innovator, I unbuckled myself while the cups were lifting off the seat trays, got up, stumbled over to the food cart, took out a can of Coke, secured the cart back in its place, and then sat back down in my seat and enjoyed the dropped jaws of people around me as I sipped my drink. To speak with Marie Forleo, everything is figureoutable but this one was close.

Ever since I told Ann this story, she checks on me before each flight and makes sure I have jelly beans in my pocket before I head to the airport. Ann's conative talent is to stabilize a situation. She is my lifesaver.

Determine Your Conative Strengths

There are different ways of determining your conative strengths. The easiest and most accurate one is by completing a Kolbe A™ Index questionnaire. You will find information on how to take it at the end of this chapter. I highly recommend taking this 36-question assessment.

Here is how you can get an indication of your conative strengths without taking a Kolbe A™ Index test. Remember that conation is action derived from instinct. Your first conscious effort to solve a problem or begin a project often indicates your dominant natural talent. You might initiate action by doing your research first, for example. I, for instance, just brainstorm possibilities before I verify my ideas by checking facts. My wife puts together a plan of attack first before reviewing data and detailed information. This makes sense to her. Why check facts if you do not know what the plan of action is and where to look? One of my clients, Christine, however, used to believe that planning anything without having all the data first did not make sense and that taking action in the absence of complete sets of data was, plainly, "stupid." Yes, she called me stupid without knowing it.

The point is that we all initiate action in our own ways, and not one is superior to another. But how we go about solving problems or implementing our ideas and projects indicates our conative strengths. Try the following exercise:

Review your empowering statements from Step 2 and write next to each one the first action you are willing to take to make it happen. For example, your statement may read, "I am still young and have the power to change into a more active lifestyle."

Now think about what this means in terms of concrete first action. There is no right or wrong answer. Just write down what you are willing to do first. Listen to your heart, not your head. If you have multiple actions in mind that you would take as first steps, then write them all down.

List what you are willing to not do. I know this is awkwardly phrased, but it's on purpose. I do want you to be clear on what you consciously won't do. You may simply not know how, or you do not like the idea of doing it, or it's "just not what you do."

Your list of nonactions may include that you won't do yoga or get up at 5 in the morning to fit exercise into your day or give up meat. Capture it all in your worksheet. When you are done, it may look like this:

TEAM LAWLESS
LEARN AND LIVE SUCCESS

Will Do / Won't Do Worksheet

Empowering Statement	Will do	Won't do
I am still young and have the power to change into a more active lifestyle.	Research physical activities that are preferred for people living with diabetes and that I like.	Get up at 5 in the morning to fit exercise into my day.

This exercise is by no means a scientific approach to determining your natural talents or conative profile. It is not an assessment tool to get clarity on your natural talents but a useful approach for defining your way of getting things done with more ease in your Diabetes Mastery™.

The surefire way of determining your natural strengths is to take a Kolbe A™ Index test. Designed by Kathy Kolbe, this instrument quantifies your natural talents and gives you the best possible understanding of your own natural instincts. It allows you to begin the process of maximizing your diabetes potential. Get it on my resource page: http://bloodsugarincheck.com.

I highly recommend that you take this assessment before you continue reading this book. I know that understanding my natural talents has helped me manage my diabetes. I am hopeful that better understanding your natural strengths will help you do the same. The exciting news is that Kathy is currently working on better understanding the way conative strengths may affect the way people handle their own diabetes care and offering suggestions on how to improve outcomes.

Until then, my "Will Do/Won't Do Worksheet" is the tool to use in your Diabetes Mastery™.

CHAPTER SEVEN

Step 4: Find Your Diabetes Flow

I am so thrilled that you have come so far in your journey to Diabetes Mastery™. Welcome to Step 4. This is where you'll start taking control of your blood sugar levels and your relationship with diabetes with concrete and constructive action.

Here is what you have accomplished so far:

In Step 1 you let all your frustrations out in a list of all the things you want to disappear from your life with diabetes. You also now understand the fears and forces that have kept these inconveniences in your life.

In Step 2 you used the Wheel of Diabetes Mastery™ to identify the one area in your life that you will focus on to keep your blood sugar in check. Focusing on this pie piece also helps you eliminate the aspects of your life that cause you to be depressed, overwhelmed, angry, worried, frustrated, sad, jealous, or pitiful. You then created statements for yourself that empower you to take action.

In Step 3 you committed to creating positive change with concrete first actions to improve your diabetes health by deciding what you will and will not do to make your diabetes life the way you want it.

Here in Step 4, you will make your action easy and natural to implement using your diabetes Flow Finder™. You will get into the flow with an exercise that helps you focus on only those tasks that keep you energized. You will dump what holds you back and do more of what keeps you moving forward with ease.

Manage Diabetes Your Way

The Flow Finder™ is an easy-to-use process that I use with my executive clients to maximize their potential at work, grow their businesses 10 times, deepen family relations and love, increase self-care, and lift their spirits high. It is the one tool that has consistently helped CEOs, business owners, and project managers alike get the results they want in business and life.

My wife, Ann, and I use the Flow Finder™ in all aspects of our lives, and it is one of the main reasons the love between us keeps on growing and why we complement each other so well.

A while back I got very stressed over filling out a form. As someone who naturally uses shortcuts, I will do everything I can to bypass bureaucracy and its forms and red tape. But sometimes, they just have to be dealt with.

This happened when we moved to Ann's home country, Ireland, and I needed to convert my German driver's license into an Irish one using my American passport. Can you already guess how terrified I was when I envisioned going through the process? It usually requires filling out forms that are wrapped in paper, which are covered in even more paper.

Not so in Ireland. It turned out that I only needed to fill out a three-page form with key information and references to essential documents, such as a letter from my doctor confirming that I was fit for driving, proof of residency, and so on.

I was not able to complete the form. I lost track of which information goes where and even confused the page sequence. I eventually threw my hands up in the air and almost surrendered to the idea that I will never have an Irish driver's license. Ann, on the other hand, who has a natural talent for organizing, laughed her head off when she saw me all animated. It took her less than 5 minutes to get the pages back in order, fill in the blanks, and then show me where I needed to sign.

On the flip side, I have the ability to simplify things and get results faster by shortcutting processes. Getting a driver's license in Ireland as an American is a lengthy and costly process that includes passing a driver theory test, applying for a learner's driving permit, and completing a driving test—even if you have driven accident free for 20 years in the US. To add insult to injury, you will need to put a big sign with a red letter N (for "new driver") on the front and rear windows of your car for a year.

I was not ready to do that, and one day I found a lifetime driver's license from more than 30 years ago in Germany that had my maiden name on it (for the record, I changed my last name to Ann's when we got married). So, off I went with my US passport, a German driver's license with a different name on it, an American marriage certificate, and my Irish green card to obtain my Irish driver's license. It worked. I needed to apply twice, because I did not have all the papers that I needed the first time around, but the authorities transferred my German license with my old name to an Irish one within 2 weeks. I have a natural ability to shortcut, and I found a legal and legitimate way of using it to get the result I wanted.

I use the same talent in my diabetes care. I do not chart and graph my blood sugar levels. I also will not log blood glucose, medication, or meals, even when an app gives me the ability to keep track easily. Other people will do that but not me. As a shortcutter, it stresses me out. I may do it for a few days and then forget about it.

I leave these tasks to technology. I use a cable to transfer my glucose levels from the meter to the app. Even better, I like to use a glucose meter that I can plug directly into my iPhone or the ones that transmit information wirelessly. The *FreeStyle Libre*, for example, is a flash glucose meter that measures, logs, analyzes, and shares my data automatically. It is blood-sugar-in-check heaven for me. The *Dexcom* is a continuous glucose meter that does the same thing in real time and also alerts you to hypos.

Unfortunately, these options are not available in all countries, and some may not be covered by your health insurance, so they are not always a viable option. But these are the shortcuts and technologies that I want to use. Equally important, I will not use any app that requires me to add information by hand systematically and frequently; I will not waste money or energy on them.

The easiest way for me to manage my blood sugar levels would be to use an insulin pump, such as the *Medtronic MiniMed*. This never fit my lifestyle, which included full contact martial arts, aggressive Rollerblading, and travel to countries where good hygiene is not always an option. The thought of having to clean and maintain a catheter, even if it's ever so tiny, has stressed me out. It's not what I naturally do well and it would only be a matter of time before I fail using the device.

Some of my friends with diabetes love and enjoy their insulin pumps and are great at using apps in their diabetes management. They thoroughly enjoy entering their weight, exercise, food intake, and glucose readings and then seeing it all charted out with trend lines and all. I, however, will only use a scale that automatically sends my weight to my iPhone app each time I step on it, and I rely on a glucose meter that analyzes my long-term results. There are only two pieces of information that I need from my devices to stay free from long-term complications. One, how close am I to a healthy weight? And two, what's the trend line for my estimated A1c?

You may need and want more information to manage your diabetes effectively or more structure than I do. You may find my approach too risky and demand more certainty.

My personal diabetes success strategy is useful only to me. But my promise to you is not to give you the one and only way to keep your blood sugar in check but instead a seven-step Diabetes Mastery™ process that helps you find an individualized solution that enables you to live a healthy and fulfilling life with your illness in collaboration with your diabetes care team.

The Flow Finder™ exercise is one vital tool in your seven-step Diabetes Mastery™ for a beautiful life. On the next page is how it works.

Target Your Diabetes Transformation

Use your completed worksheet from Step 3 that lists all the actions that you will and won't take, and then transfer them to the Diabetes Transformation Target™.

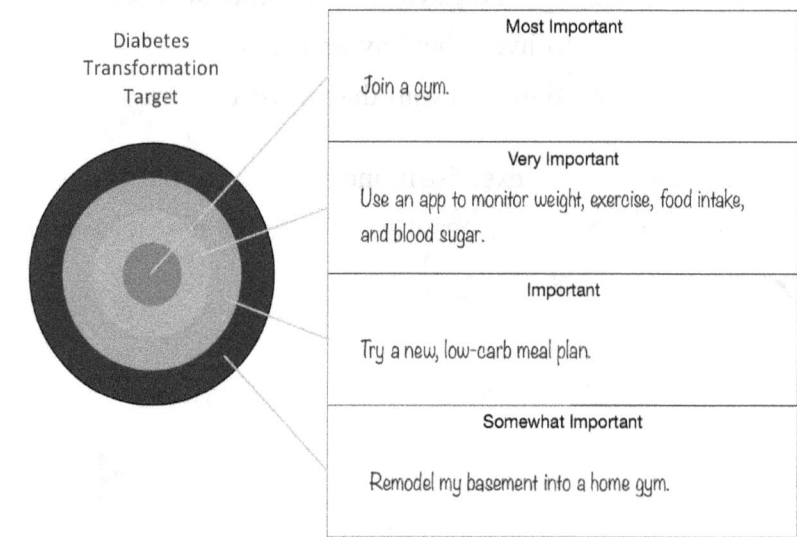

TEAM LAWLESS
LEARN AND LIVE SUCCESS

Diabetes Transformation Target

Most Important
Join a gym.
Very Important
Use an app to monitor weight, exercise, food intake, and blood sugar.
Important
Try a new, low-carb meal plan.
Somewhat Important
Remodel my basement into a home gym.

© 2017 – 2018 Andrew Lawless and Rockant, Inc

Do not write more than one task per circle. In the beginning, everything that you have in your head seems überimportant. This exercise is meant to give you clarity. So, you will need to make some hard decisions.

If you have too many balls in the air, then you will drop them all. Four tasks or projects is a healthy number to remember. Biologically, your brain cannot process more than seven commitments at the same time, plus or minus two. In an average person, the synapses are well-suited to handle about four. After that, it gets hard. If you have more than four tasks, then we will need to park the remaining ones for another time.

Get Your Diabetes Flow Factor™

Once you have targeted your tasks, turn to your Flow Factor™ Worksheet. In this step, you will determine the value (aka Flow Factor™) you bring to each task. You can download the full-size worksheet on the resource page for this book at http://bloodsugarincheck.com. If you need help completing this worksheet, email me at andrew@bloodsugarincheck.com.

TEAM LAWLESS
LEARN AND LIVE SUCCESS

Flow Factor Worksheet

Task	Talent	Motivation	Expertise	Flow Factor

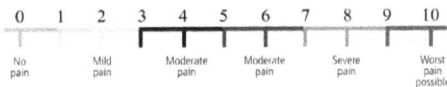

0 1 2 3 4 5 6 7 8 9 10

No pain | Mild pain | Moderate pain | Moderate pain | Severe pain | Worst pain possible

© 2012 - 2018 Andrew Lawless and Rockant, Inc.

In the next step, you will rate each task based on your talent, whether or not you like the task, and if you have the knowledge, judgment, and experience to perform it successfully. You will give every task a rating from 1 to 10 in each category. A score of 1 means that it is easy and painless for you, and 10 means performing this task would cause you excruciating pain. Do the following:

- In the "Talent" column, rate how easy this task comes to you. I am sure that you have a talent that your friends, colleagues, and family members know you have. They may even come to you for advice on a regular basis because of this talent, but you might not think of it as something special because it comes so easily to you. Rate how easy it is for you to perform this task. Do not confuse this rating with whether or not you look forward to performing it. You will rate that in the next column.

  As an example, sorting socks may come easily to you, but you may not like doing it.

Your Flow Factor™ Worksheet should look now like this:

Flow Factor Worksheet

Task	Talent	Motivation	Expertise	Flow Factor
Walk around the block each day.	0			
Research gyms in my area.	7			
Hire a babysitter for when I am at the gym.	4			
Use an online app for diabetes management.	2			
Cook plant based meals.	6			

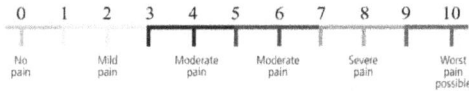

```
0   1   2   3   4   5   6   7   8   9   10
No      Mild    Moderate  Moderate  Severe    Worst
pain    pain    pain      pain      pain      pain
                                              possible
```

© 2012 - 2018 Andrew Lawless and Rockant, Inc.

- Now go to the next column, "Motivation," and rate how much you enjoy performing the task. This should be easy for you, because we often have a pretty good idea of what we like and don't like. We have spent a whole lifetime figuring that out. If you are really excited, then your pain level is low; if it feels like someone is pulling your teeth out, then your pain level is closer to 10.

For example, I have the talent to find the fastest way to a sports game, but as someone who has no interest in watching sports whatsoever, the thought of wasting my time in a ballpark makes me cringe. So, while my talent in helping my family get there is high, my motivation for joining them is low. I'd rather have dinner with them afterward and do something that is more meaningful while they enjoy watching their team.

- In the "Expertise" column, rate whether you have the knowledge, experience, or judgment to complete the task. If you have all the knowledge and expertise in the world, then it should be easy for you to perform the task, but if you have, no clue where to start, then you are probably at a pain level of 10 because it will take you tremendous effort to acquire the proficiency that the task requires.

Finally, summarize your score across each line.

Your Flow Factor™ Worksheet should now look like this:

TEAM LAWLESS
LEARN AND LIVE SUCCESS

Flow Factor Worksheet

Task	Talent	Motivation	Expertise	Flow Factor
Walk around the block each day.	0	0	0	0
Research gyms in my area.	7	10	10	27
Hire a babysitter for when I am at the gym.	4	6	5	15
Use an online app for diabetes management.	2	0	7	9
Cook plant based meals.	6	8	8	18

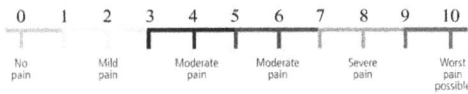

0	1	2	3	4	5	6	7	8	9	10
No pain		Mild pain		Moderate pain		Moderate pain		Severe pain		Worst pain possible

© 2012 - 2018 Andrew Lawless and Rockant, Inc.

Do, Doctor, Delegate or Dump

You have now rated how much each task fits into your unique way of getting things done. Two people can have the same list of tasks but completely different ratings. It is not important how you compare with others. What counts is that you were honest with yourself.

These ratings determine how you will get things done. You should see scores between 0 and 30 in the "Flow Factor" column.

Here is what they mean.

0 - 9: Do

Each task with a score between 1 and 9 keeps you in flow. You have all the talent to perform the task, you like doing it, and you have the knowledge, judgment, and experience to get the results you want. Go for it. You have the highest chance of successfully completing this task.

10 - 20: Doctor

The tasks with scores in this range are the ones that I spend most of my time helping my clients with in coaching sessions. The objective is to doctor these tasks in a way that they can easily be either completed, delegated, dumped, or automated with technology. Ideally, you should not have any tasks in this category, although this is not always possible. It is inevitable that you will find yourself doing some things that are not a great fit for you, but you'll want to keep them to a manageable minimum.

I find solutions for my clients in 90% of all cases. Take the "hire a babysitter" task from my example above. I have sufficient motivation, affection, and knowledge to complete the task. But my wife, Ann, can do it more efficiently. So, instead of doing it myself, I ask her if she could take it on. In this case, I delegate to the task to Ann.

In another example, monitoring your blood sugar may entirely be in your range of capabilities, but you may hate entering results into your app because they are already captured in your glucose meter. This is an easy fix. You could drop the manual entry by using a glucose meter that wirelessly transfers your results to your app or use a continuous glucose monitoring system. Task dumped.

21 - 30: Delegate or Dump

You will not provide any value to tasks that have a total score between 21 and 30. You have neither the conative talent, the motivation, nor sufficient knowledge, judgment, and experience to get positive results.

That leaves you with three choices to dump them.

1.   Delegate the task to someone else.

2.   Find a technology solution.

3.   Don't do it at all and be fine with it.

Before you continue to the next step, take the same approach for each task on your list.

It will take you longer in the beginning to use this worksheet. Think of it as learning how to drive a car. First, you learn the theory and the rules of the road. Then a driving instructor teaches you how to actually drive. Learning how to change gears, change lanes, watch the traffic around you at all times, and anticipate what the driver in front of you will do requires you to stay fully engaged when you start out. But after 3 weeks, you perform all of these tasks so automatically that you can have a conversation at the same time.

The same will happen with your Flow Factor™ and Flow Finder™. When Ann and I started using this way of planning our lives, we needed to think about how we go about each task individually and as a couple. Today, it flows naturally between Ann and me.

When we go on a road trip, for example, she is the one who makes sure we have snacks and bottles of water in the car, have enough cash on hand for paying tolls, and know where to stop for breaks. She has the natural strength to organize (her talent), is excited to go on a road trip with Dylan and me (motivation), and knows exactly what to do (experience). She even has a process in place to get this done.

I, too, am thrilled about spending a quality day with my family and exploring a new area, city, or country (motivation). And I am the one who has the natural strength to get us to our destination on time without stressing (talent) and find other fun things to do on the way that were not initially in our plans (experience).

As with all power couples, we have become interdependent and hardly need to discuss who does what anymore. We just do it without thinking about it. The same will happen to you if you consistently use the Flow Factor™ Worksheet for at least 3 weeks. You will then begin to naturally use the Flow Finder™ without having to fill out the Flow Factor™ Worksheet anymore.

After you have completed your Flow Finder™ Worksheet, you will have successfully created a strategy for your personal Diabetes Mastery™ in a way that works for you. Now schedule an appointment with your diabetes care team to discuss and finalize your plans. Do not make decisions about your medical care without the consent of your doctors. They are essential contributors to your long-term well-being. Consult them for all your choices.

In the next step, you will condition yourself to stick with your finalized diabetes management strategy and change your relationship with your illness forever.

CHAPTER EIGHT

Step 5: Condition Yourself for Blood Sugar Success

How cool is that? With just a few exercises, you have created total clarity on what you need to do to get your blood sugar in check. You may be surprised that your first focus area is not diabetes management but one of the other six pie pieces in your Wheel of Diabetes Mastery™.

At this point, you should feel very excited about your action plan, and it should be easy for you to implement it. But there is a catch.

You will still need to follow the advice of your diabetes care team. You may still have to prick your fingers and take your medication multiple times a day. You will continue to collaborate closely with your family physician, endocrinologist, and other doctors for your eye care, kidney health, heart disease prevention, or foot care, for example.

They may eventually find something that discourages or

depresses you, such as a blockage in your arteries, nerve damage, or diabetes-related vision loss. Your A1c results will not always reflect the hard work you have put in. You will have mornings when your blood sugar is inexplicably high, even though you did everything right the day before.

In these moments, it is easy to give up and feel downtrodden. Why bother? All this work for what? Know that it is absolutely OK to be in this lousy state. We are a moody species. Sadness, anger, and disappointment have always been a part of the human experience. Bad moods are typical responses to the challenges that life throws at us. That happens by design.

Feeling sad or being in a foul mood helps us focus on our situation and increases our ability to find a solution. It reduces distractions, such as irrelevant, false, or misleading information. Our judgment improves during those moments, and people who are sad ask more questions and produce better answers to solve their problems. A mild bad mood causes people to treat others less selfishly and more fairly. Sadness can also enhance compassion and trigger creative action, such as expressing your feelings in a poem, a picture, or a song.

Clinical depression and never-ending intense sadness are obviously severe conditions that require professional help and intervention. Bruce Springsteen, one of the most creative and successful songwriters in history, famously wrote about his battle with depression in his *New York Times* best seller *Born to Run*. But many people who claim they are depressed may just "feel depressed," and it is a temporary response to a challenging or difficult situation. They are signaling to friends and family that they need help, because people are often more willing to help when they know that their loved ones feel down.

All emotions, not just negative ones, are alarm signals that ask us to be more attentive and prompt us to take action. When we are attracted to someone, the call to action is to walk over and introduce ourselves. When we love something, it is to nurture it. Negative emotions are calls to action just as much.

Frustration signals that you are doing the same thing over and over again and expecting a different result. You will need to change your approach to achieving your goals. For example, you may drink a lot of diet soda because, in your mind, it is free of calories free, carbohydrates, and sugar. But the artificial sweeteners also confuse your body, because they taste sweet but don't provide calories, which messes with your metabolism. Giving up diet soda and drinking more water may be the key to getting better results.

Disappointment tells you that your expectations are not being met or an outcome that you anticipated won't happen. Therefore, you will need to change your expectations. For example, maybe your timeframe for lowering your A1c or losing weight is too short.

Anger is typically a sign that you have been wronged. Someone—or even you—broke an important rule of yours, and you are upset. Your rule may be that life is just and you think that it is unfair that you have diabetes while other people are healthy. Your standards might not match reality, so you will need to change them, unless you want to stay angry until you die. Life is not supposed to be fair. The universe throws us challenges because it wants us to learn and grow. Anger is a call to clarify or change your rules and maybe even your view of how life should be.

If you stay angry and won't learn, then you will eventually burn out and seek "freedom" from diabetes by neglecting the basics of managing it. All negative emotions can quickly derail your new plans to keep your blood sugar in check and your A1c down. Your focus will then promptly shift to all the negative things that diabetes has introduced into your life.

As you learned in Step 1, where focus goes, energy flows, and you will invite more negativity into your life if you focus on the negative. Having negative thoughts is normal, but you are not supposed to stay in them. Your job is to understand the signals that emotions send you and act accordingly. Once you understand the message, you can do something about it.

The moment you have interpreted the signal, you can find the root cause that makes you feel that way. Finding the right solution to eliminate the cause, however, requires you to be in a better state of mind. Think about it: When was the last time you were anxious about a crisis at home or at work, pressed your fingertips into the creases of your forehead, tried to come up with a great solution, and actually found one? It does not happen. You rarely have a great idea in a lousy state.

When was the last time a completely new idea or alternative to a preconceived solution popped in your head? It was probably during a shower, a walk on the beach, a hike in the mountains, a yoga class, or another moment where you were in a positive state of mind, away from distractions.

This is also why I advise my coaching clients to leave their smart watches and phones in a locker when they go to yoga class or at home when they walk in nature or spend quality time with family. You do not need constant notifications unless someone in your family or circle of friends is giving birth, just went into or came out of surgery, or is dying. The reason so many people have their best ideas in the shower is because this is the rare moment when they are free from distractions. The idea of writing this book came to me while walking the Billy Goat Trail along the Potomac River near Washington, D.C.

Change Your Focus, Change Your Emotions

You need to be in a positive mental state to make effective changes. In a negative mental state, it is easy to believe that you cannot do anything to make it better. Remember what you told yourself the last time you were newly in love. There is nothing that you cannot do when you are in love and feel deep gratitude for this new person in your life. Clients tell me that they can do anything when they are in love. And I bet that is true for you too.

I am also sure you remember the first time someone broke your heart. These are the moments when your sense of self-worth is practically zero. You tell yourself that you are not good enough, that life is miserable, that men are pigs or women are mean. Everything in life at that moment sucks, and it is hard to envision yourself being loved by someone new.

If you have ever had a painful breakup and are now married to the love of your life, then you also now know that the breakup happened for a reason. But the question that I want to ask you is, how is it that one day you think you are the greatest and the next, you think you are the dried-up scum between the dirt and the bottom of your trash can? You are the same person on both days.

What changed is your focus on life and your beliefs about yourself. One day you are focused on the beauty and glory of love; the next, on the pain. Your emotions are formed by your focus and beliefs.

If you believe that diabetes is a curse, then you are right. If you think that you will never be able to manage your diabetes and get your blood sugar levels in check, then your brain will find a way to validate your belief. If you reckon you have the liberty to be angry and disappointed, then you are also correct. You will kick your reticular activating system into high gear to filter out everything else that does not fit your belief, which will inundate you with more evidence that you have the right to be angry, disappointed, hurt, dejected, and depressed.

If, on the other hand, you believe that diabetes is a gift, an opportunity to grow, a force to drive you farther than you ever thought you would go, or the universe's way of telling you that you need to learn, then you are also correct.

Yes, you can feel like a failure when you wake up in the morning and your blood sugar is still high, even if you managed your food intake, medication, and exercise by the book the day before. Alternatively, you can ask yourself, *What can I learn from this experience?*

Success is a matter of massive action, which, in turn, is the result of experience, and experience often comes from failure. Each time you fail, you can tell yourself how much you suck, or you can say to yourself that you are one step closer to your goal. Change your focus, change your emotions. The choice is yours.

Change Your Language, Change Your Blood Sugar

What you say to yourself changes how you feel. Telling yourself that you are bad at organizing makes you feel inadequate, while telling yourself that you have a fantastic ability to shortcut processes makes you proud. Both thoughts state the same thing, but they cause different emotions and actions. When you think of yourself as a lousy organizer, you may eventually submit to living in chaos. But believing that you excel at shortcutting makes you want to find more opportunities to get the order and organization you want in life faster.

By the way, just in case you happen to be good at organizing, we shortcutters could easily say that you make a complicated thing more complicated. It is all a matter of focus and belief and the words we use.

How you describe yourself changes how you feel. Likewise, the words you use to describe your diabetes define how you think about it and what action you are going to take.

When I read through posts on Facebook groups, diabetes forums, and blogs, I see two different ways of describing the disease. Group 1 posts statements such as:

"It sucks ass."

"Hurricane, tornado, whirlwind, roller coaster ride, tsunami, volcano!"

"Annoying, head trip, and so expensive."

"Yes…it's a daily struggle."

"It's exhausting!"

"I hate this disease."

Group 2 displays a different attitude:

"I don't see it as a battle. It's about having a management plan that works most of the time."

"It's the hand I was dealt...gotta play it through."

"Always a fighter, never a victim!"

"I decide how I live my life, not diabetes."

"Good, bad, who is really normal?"

"It's what was given, so I deal with it."

"Check sugar, adjust insulin, enjoy life. Repeat."

"Whether high, low, or perfect glucose, I manage it and live my life."

I find it quite interesting that the people in the second group generally appear to have their blood sugar in check, while the first group does not. My question is whether the first group is dejected because their blood sugar is uncontrollable or if they are having a hard time managing their blood sugar because of the stories they are telling themselves about their illness.

In Step 1 of your diabetes transformation process, I shared how Alicia Crum's research gave us good answers to this question. We learned that believing that our work is consistent with a healthy lifestyle is enough to lower our blood pressure. Words matter.

One of the terms that bothers me the most in diabetes care is "blood sugar control." It presupposes that people with diabetes can control their blood sugar to stay at normal levels. We cannot. Our bodies sometimes have their own minds, and no matter what we do, we cannot exercise control. I mean this literally.

Your heart started beating in your mother's womb before your brain had fully developed. Something made that heart beat, and it might as well mess with your blood sugar now and then when it wants to. In addition, your Wheel of Diabetes Mastery™ has shown you that several outside factors, such as finances, family support, spirituality, and other constraints, may take your control over your blood sugar levels away from you.

When you say to yourself that you have "poor control" over your blood sugar, you are judging yourself on a standard of perfection that can never be achieved. You will always feel like a failure and eventually come to the conclusion that you have no power over your life in general. Instead of obsessing over blood sugar control, strive for the power to keep it in check.

We know from medical studies that negative words release cortisol in patients after abdominal surgeries and make morphine less effective for pain management. People drink significantly more alcohol after hearing negative words. Calling people "obese" and "fat" makes them feel lousy about themselves and, as a result, they often continue eating junk food and won't go back to a healthy lifestyle that would enable them to lose weight.

In people with diabetes, negative words trigger a stress response that can lead to high blood glucose levels, inflammation, and a weakened immune system. Equally important, they contribute to diabetes distress, which increases A1c and decreases motivation to push yourself to higher levels of health.

We hear terms like "obese," "low blood sugar control," and "poor medication adherence" from health care professionals all the time. One report by a doctor of mine once stated that I "failed to achieve adequate glycemic control" during my recovery from knee surgery, as if that would somehow make me feel better and accelerate healing. But in the end, these are microaggressions at best. That's just the way some doctors speak. It does not make it right, but I also do not allow these statements to faze me.

The words that hurt the most are the ones we say to ourselves. That little but constant voice in our heads is our worst critic and enemy. It constantly tells us that we are not good enough, that diabetes is the worst thing that could have ever happened to us, that we will never be able to deal with it, or that life is going to be terrible. In the end, it is we who believe we are a burden to others and do not actively involve family and friends in our care.

Yes, there are always assholes that will bring you down. But will you actually measure your self-worth against words from a moron? You cannot change an idiot, but you can change what you say to yourself.

Nothing anyone ever says to you hurts you. It is the story that you make up behind those words that upsets you. I used to have a client in defensive tactics who called me, and I quote, "motherfucker." That was the biggest compliment I could have hoped for, coming from a person who once told me that his gun was jammed by saying, "This fucking fucker is fucking fucked." I was not upset at all. I knew his words were expressions of appreciation. I felt honored and respected. The same words from a random person on the street could have easily upset me, because I would have interpreted them differently.

Nothing in this world has meaning until you give it one. Diabetes can make you a stronger fighter or a weaker victim. It can "suck ass" or it can "be a challenge." It is your choice, and you will make it here in this chapter.

Change the Meaning of Diabetes and Make It Stick

For me, diabetes has always been a blessing. I firmly believe that this is the reason I am free from even minor complications after having lived with it for more than 40 years. I have rarely looked at the danger of my illness and always had my eye on the possibilities it brings. In my teens, I used to be more responsible and reliable than many of my schoolmates, because managing my blood sugar instilled discipline in me and held me accountable for my actions early on in life. I did not have to go to mandatory military service in Germany and instead was able to focus on an exciting career 2 years earlier than most of my friends.

If you are dwelling on negative thoughts, or at least more often than you should, and allow them to linger, then you are at risk of first neglecting and then ditching your action plan that you developed in Step 4. Just remember how many New Year's resolutions you have given up on in your life. If you are like most people, then it took you less than 3 weeks to break them. Knowing which changes you want to make is easy but following through on them is hard.

I am here to keep you on track to Diabetes Mastery™. Most people don't follow through on their promises to themselves, because they associate their goals, their situation, or the process of achieving results with a negative experience. Take, for example, going on an alkaline diet. Not being able to eat meat and munching primarily on water-based vegetables is the definition of hell for carnivores. If these are your feelings about your new food choices, then you will not make it through the first few days, during which you'll feel hungry and fart and pee a lot. Your cravings for the fullness in your belly that come from a big, juicy steak will overpower your desire to live a long, healthy life. Sounds crazy, but that's how your brain and mind work.

When you keep associating your plan with negative experiences, you will not follow through. When people associate quitting smoking with gaining weight, they will not succeed. After the financial crisis of 2008–2009, many Americans stopped investing in the stock market, because they associated investing their money with loss and ultimately missed out on the longest bull market in history. If they had invested in an S&P 500 Index about 9 months after the crash, their savings would have tripled by now—excluding compound interest.

I do not want you to lose out on your investment in yourself and your health in favor of that ice cream today, the fun at the BBQ tomorrow, or the business presentation next week. You will instead form new associations between your plans and your feelings about them. The process is called neuro-associative conditioning (NAC), a science that was developed by Tony Robbins, a best-selling author, philanthropist, and life coach who has changed the destiny of millions of people.

I mentioned NAC earlier, in Step 2 of your Diabetes Mastery™ process. We are finally at the point where you will use it for your benefit. To change your life with diabetes, you must link pleasure to your new choice and then experience gratification over and over, until it becomes a habit. That is the only way to make it stick and for you to follow through.

To begin the process, write down the following for each of your new actions and plans from Step 4:

1. Three benefits you will gain by taking this action or step

2. Three emotional reasons you must take this action or step

3. Three ways in which you can enjoy taking this action

Use the worksheet below. Here is an example of what an entry could look like:

TEAM LAWLESS
LEARN AND LIVE SUCCESS

Positive Association Worksheet

Action / Step	3 Benefits	3 Reasons	3 Ways I Can Enjoy This
Practice yoga 3 times a week.	Strengthens my heart.	Want to be alive for my kids' weddings.	Buddy up with my son.
	Increases my energy.	Need to see the pyramids of Egypt before I die.	Spa day after each successful week
	Weight loss.	Want to be able to throw balls with grandchildren.	Buy nice yoga outfits.

The first column is called "3 Benefits." This is self-explanatory. Just list what you want to result from your actions. This may be better heart health, lower A1c, increased energy, more money, less weight, and so on.

Pay particular attention to the next column, "3 Reasons." List here all the emotional reasons you need to act now. Do not just write down a statement that reads like "makes me feel better." Be specific.

Let me explain the importance of this column in a little bit more with diet plans. The reasons people want to lose weight are typically specific. Maybe they want to be able to climb up stairs without huffing and puffing, look sexier, or kick a soccer ball around with their grandchildren without risking a heart attack.

The same is true for making money. The dollar bills alone are not the reason. They do not make anyone happier. It is the lifestyle or the experiences that money can buy that people want, such as being able to see the world, no longer worrying about paying bills, or just being admired as a success in one's community.

In the "3 Ways I Can Enjoy This" column, list all the rewards you can give yourself. You can team up with someone to both hold each other accountable and deepen your friendship or relationship. One of my clients, for instance, takes her grown-up daughter to yoga class. This way, they pursue a mutual new interest, and after each class, they catch up on their lives over a green smoothie or almond butter protein shake. You can bet that she has never missed a single class, even at times when she doesn't really feel like going.

As an example of successful NAC, I am sharing with you my approach to quitting alcohol. I listed the following three benefits:

1. More energy throughout the day

2. Saving $300 a month not spent on wine

3. Two more hours a day for self-improvement and personal development

Knowing that I would be easily tempted by a glass of Barolo or a decent gin and tonic, I listed next to each statement a reason that was higher than myself:

I will have enough energy to spend quality time with my son Dylan at night, rather than melting into my couch. I do not want to regret missing the opportunity to experience him while he is still young.

I want Dylan to leave my house with savings that give him a kick-start for a new life when he arrives at that point.

I need to be a role model for both my older and younger sons, Arian and Dylan, respectively, so they keep on growing to their best selves as they age.

I figured that just sipping on a glass of wine would be synonymous with giving up on my sons. I have not had one since.

I used the last column of the Positive Association Worksheet as my insurance policy. By making it fun, I ensured I would stay away from alcohol when it gets hard.

One of the problems with giving up drinking, for example, is that many people assume that you have a drinking problem. Some will silently label you as a recovering alcoholic; others will plainly ask you about Alcoholics Anonymous or ask you if you suffer from alcoholism. It can be quite difficult to reject a drink. So, it was important for me to make the rejection fun. I researched a few responses that leave people stunned, and each time I use them, I crack up when I see their puzzled faces.

In addition, each week that I successfully kept alcohol out of my body, I rewarded myself with a treat, such as watching a movie, eating artisanal chocolate, buying a small gadget, or spending extra time in the gym. Once every 3 months, I'd reward myself with something bigger, such as a massage or an item for the house that continues to remind me of my success.

This last column in your Positive Association Worksheet helps you decide in advance how you will reward yourself.

Enjoy making these new neuro-associative connections. Make even the process of writing them down pleasurable. Put your favorite music on, have a cup of tea, or go to your favorite place—a coffee shop, a park, your favorite room in the house— when you complete this worksheet. The more you are in a positive state of mind when you write, the better.

When you are done, read this list every day. Take it with you whenever you can. Constant reminders, along with rewards, are great ways of reinforcing your new habits.

CHAPTER NINE

Step 6: Overcome Unconstructive Blood Sugar Management Patterns

You have made so much progress by now. You are absolutely amazing. Just think about how far you have come. You went from struggling with keeping your blood sugar in check to committing to action and making sure that you feel good and motivated about it. That is huge. I am so proud of you.

Did you know that 90% of people who buy self-help books never implement what they have learned? But not you. The fact that you are reading this chapter tells me that you are amongst the 10% of achievers. Most people fail because they stop following their dreams and abandon their action plans too early. But you have stuck with your plans. Wow. I am so grateful that you have followed me so far, and I am equally thrilled that you continue to make progress.

You are not quite over the hill yet though. There is one more hurdle you need to jump, one more mind trick you need to play on your brain. This organ in your head is quite complex and not ready to give up yet, pulling you back into your old habits. The region in your brain that is responsible for this attempted regress is called the basal ganglia. It is a group of structures with multiple functions. One of them is to store your routines and rituals so that the brain is freed from performing repetitive tasks and you can act without thinking. The problem is that these habits are like bed bugs; once they are there, it is hard to get rid of them.

Have you ever wanted to visit a friend on a Sunday morning and drove to your office instead? That is an example of your basal ganglia in action, and it is usually helpful. The basal ganglia put you on autopilot and enable you to drive the car while having a conversation. They help you cook while listening to the radio and get dressed in the morning while you think about what outcomes you want for your day. In short, the basal ganglia make you more effective by storing repetitive tasks so that you can perform them without thinking.

The downside is that once your habits are programmed into your brain, they are hard to change. Your driving to the office on a Sunday morning was not intentional. You set out with the goal of driving to your friend's house, but at one point in time, your basal ganglia quietly took over and made you go where you always drive and not to the destination you wanted.

The same will happen with your new plans for managing your diabetes. The old programming in your brain will want you to do what you have always done, and quite often you are not even aware of it. Look at your morning routines, for example. Do you wake up and first take a shower before you have breakfast? Or do you have a cup of coffee and then soap up? I would guess that you follow the same sequence every day without thinking about it. You probably also wash the same armpit first when you shower. How do I know? Because we all do it.

What rituals and habits have you adopted? Do you routinely skip lunch at work because you are too busy and then later have an all-out feast that spikes your blood sugar? Do you snack at night in front of the TV and lose track of how many carbs you ate? What do you do when you come home from a stressful day at work? Do you open a bottle of wine and keep sipping too much of the good stuff, which also makes your blood sugar plummet at night? What are the issues that make you sweat the small stuff, which triggers a stress response that elevates your blood sugar?

These habits once served you in some way. Opening a bottle of wine may have been a social thing to do when meeting new friends. The small issues you sweat were once important and needed your immediate attention. Skipping lunch at work helped you finish your presentation, which aced the client meeting in the afternoon. But these routines now no longer serve you, because they worsen your blood sugar management.

Some of your rituals may even still serve you in the short run but damage your health over time and lead to complications. What, for example, do you do when you are having a hypo? Do you go to the freezer and look for ice cream and overeat? Or do you grab a few jelly beans that you have prepared in small portions to avoid putting all those extra calories and carbohydrates in your body, so you don't gain weight in the long term and cause your blood sugar to swing into the other extreme?

If you do not break your unconstructive routines, then your best-laid plans for managing your diabetes will falter. The key to making your plans successful is to identify and then change the triggers that kick your habits, routines, and rituals. One of my triggers for eating chocolate, for example, is boredom. When I am busy and moving around, I hardly ever crave sweets. But the moment I sit still and nothing much is going on, my brain asks for more variety. At those moments, I walk into the kitchen to get a piece of chocolate. But it does not stop there. I tend to continue to raid the chocolate drawer until I remember—or my iPhone reminds me of—a nearing deadline for handing in my work to a client. I then go into overdrive and finish the project without once needing something sweet.

Your Crazy and Healthy Figure Eights

I used to have two triggers for my chocolate addiction: 1. Boredom made me want chocolate. 2. A reminder of a looming deadline got my mind off it. These two triggers kept me in a crazy figure eight, a concept from the coaching methodology strategic intervention. It describes how people get stuck in habitual patterns. I have illustrated my past chocolate addictions in the graphic below:

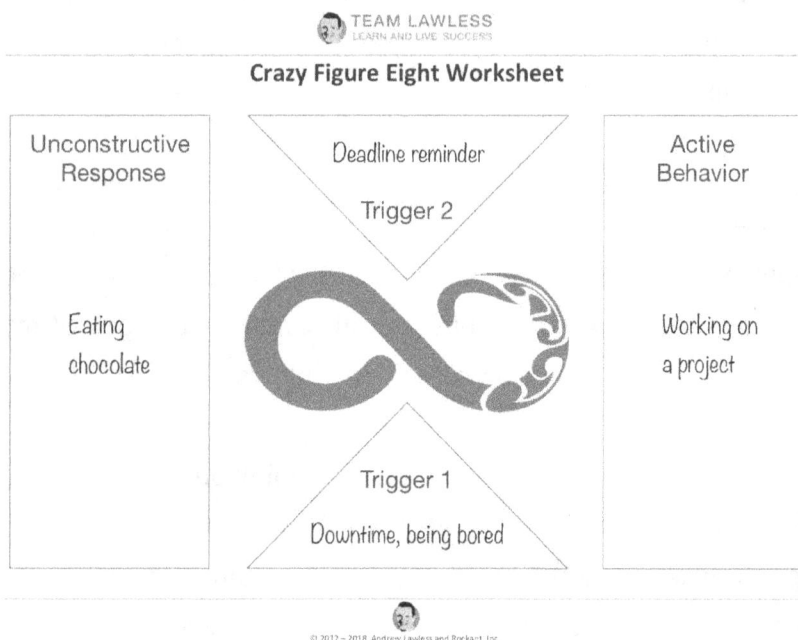

TEAM LAWLESS
LEARN AND LIVE SUCCESS

Crazy Figure Eight Worksheet

Unconstructive Response	Deadline reminder	Active Behavior
	Trigger 2	
Eating chocolate		Working on a project
	Trigger 1	
	Downtime, being bored	

© 2012 – 2018 Andrew Lawless and Rockant, Inc.

The key to breaking my chocolate addiction was to identify the triggers in the crazy eight. That was not as easy as it sounds, because once this routine had been programmed into my basal ganglia, I operated on autopilot. I had to rely on my wife, Ann, to observe that every time I was bored, I became restless and walked into the kitchen. Other people are often much better at detecting our own patterns.

Once we understand our triggers, we need to replace our unconstructive responses. Eating chocolate is not healthy. It spikes my blood sugar, contributes to weight gain, and causes plaque in my arteries because of the dairy and fat in it. My job now is to interrupt the pattern and introduce a new response. For example, I now brush my teeth instead of grabbing a piece of chocolate. My healthy figure eight looks like this:

TEAM LAWLESS
LEARN AND LIVE SUCCESS

Healthy Figure Eight Worksheet

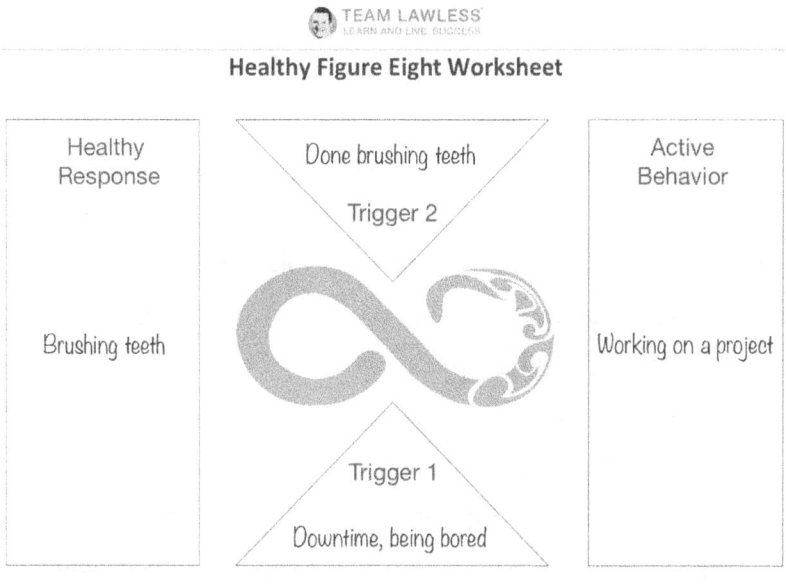

Healthy Response	Done brushing teeth	Active Behavior
	Trigger 2	
Brushing teeth		Working on a project
	Trigger 1	
	Downtime, being bored	

© 2012 – 2018 Andrew Lawless and Ruckant, Inc

Build Your Healthy Figure Eight

To build your own healthy habits, you need to reverse engineer your crazy figure eight to find trigger 1 on the bottom of the worksheet. Take the following steps:

In the "Unconstructive Response" box on the left, write down the unhealthy behavior you want to avoid. In my example, it was eating chocolate. In your case it might be drinking wine, watching television, being defensive, withdrawing from family, consciously keeping your blood sugar high, or spending too much money on shopping. Whatever unhealthy behavior you have, write it down. Only use one worksheet per unhealthy behavior that you want to avoid.

Now, remember what happened right before you started your unhealthy behavior. What was the event or circumstance that caused your action? In my example, it was boredom that triggered my going to the kitchen and searching for chocolate. For a client of mine who was a very sociable and likable woman, it was being called out for mistakes she made at work that made her very defensive. What specific event or circumstance triggers your unhealthy response? They are typically always the same. Maybe you just came home from a stressful day at work, your significant other did not empty the dishwasher, you just remembered overdue bills, your blood sugar dropped, you saw something on TV, or you just measured your glucose levels. Whatever it is, write it down in the triangle on the bottom under "Trigger 1".

Note what you were doing well right before trigger 1 switched you into unhealthy behavior. In my example, I was simply doing my job. What active behavior were you showing? Maybe you had a busy day at work or were out having a good time at a restaurant with friends. It could have been an intense workout or yoga session or an engaging conversation. Maybe you cooked or cleaned the kitchen, balanced your bank account, got dressed, or simply woke up. Write it in the "Active Behavior" box on the right side of your worksheet.

Last, identify trigger 2. Most of us do not stay in an unhealthy behavior all the time. We tend to snap out of it. My client who is defensive at work is the sweetest and most patient mother at home. I used to overeat chocolate but also craved healthy salads and smoothies, and there were times when I could not stand the smell of chocolate. Some triggers can be panic or fear. We suddenly realize that we need to be proactive about our A1c levels not to die early or experience long-term complications—and then get into gear.

When those triggers and your responses to them occur regularly, you have formed a habit that does not serve you. You are in a crazy figure eight. A particularly severe figure eight for a person with diabetes looks like this:

- Trigger 1: Blood sugar drops

- Unconstructive Response: Overeat ice cream

- Trigger 2: Blood sugar rises

- Active Behavior: Inject aggressive dose of insulin

Crazy Figure Eight Worksheet

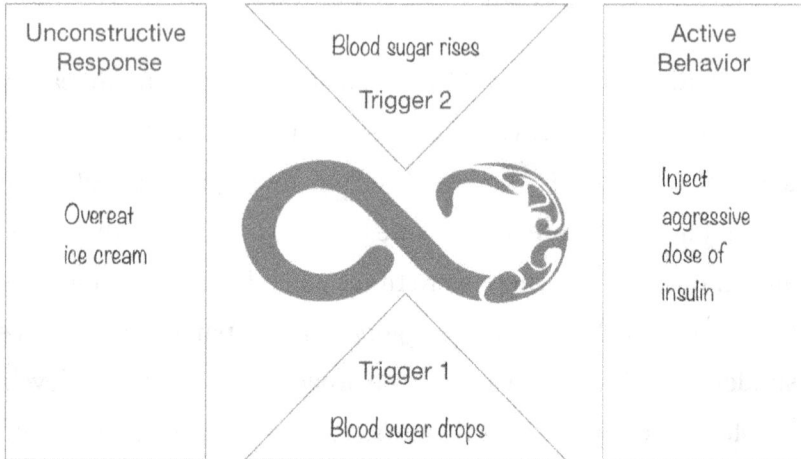

Unconstructive Response	Blood sugar rises / Trigger 2	Active Behavior
Overeat ice cream		Inject aggressive dose of insulin
	Trigger 1 / Blood sugar drops	

To turn your crazy figure eight into a healthy one, you will need to replace the unconstructive response with a healthy response that gives you the same results. In the example above, instead of eating ice cream, which also makes you gain weight, the person could have eaten jelly beans. We typically do not need more than 15 grams of carbohydrates when we have a hypo, but it takes a while for the brain to recognize when we have had enough food. So, we tend to shove carbs into our mouths until we feel better, only to realize an hour later that our blood sugar has skyrocketed.

Having prepacked bags or small containers can counteract the tendency to overeat during a hypo. The small portions remind us to contain ourselves by keeping the right number of jelly beans handy, which amounts to 15 grams of carbohydrates. Depending on the brand, that amounts to 10 to 20 jelly beans. Check the nutrition label.

When I have a hypo, I eat one pack of jelly beans and then wait 15 minutes before I recheck my blood sugar level. If it is still low, I eat another portion of jelly beans and repeat the process every 15 minutes until my blood sugar is back to normal.

TEAM LAWLESS
LEARN AND LIVE SUCCESS

Healthy Figure Eight Worksheet

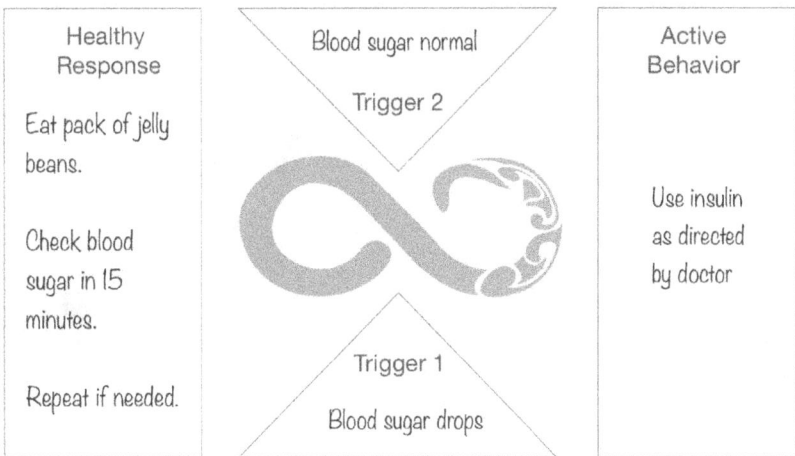

Healthy Response	Blood sugar normal	Active Behavior
Eat pack of jelly beans.	Trigger 2	Use insulin as directed by doctor
Check blood sugar in 15 minutes.		
Repeat if needed.	Trigger 1	
	Blood sugar drops	

© 2012 – 2018 Andrew Lawless and Rockwill, Inc.

You may need to use different intervals or eat fewer or more carbohydrates. Make decisions about your diabetes management in collaboration with your diabetes care team. Every person with diabetes is unique and has different needs and health care requirements.

Breaking crazy figure eights is a lifelong process. Bad habits tend to sneak in. So, enjoy the process, and see if you can even make it fun and enjoyable to involve all members of your diabetes care team. I am sure they, too, have crazy figure eights.

CHAPTER TEN

Step 7: Embrace Your Diabetes Lifestyle

Technically, you completed your diabetes transformation planning at the end of Step 6. You now have all the insights and tools to develop a mindset that enables you to keep your blood sugar in check. After going through all the exercises in this book, you have created a crystal-clear strategy and set priorities for creating a beautiful life with diabetes. You have eliminated past behavior that prevented you from succeeding and conditioned yourself to stay motivated to follow through on your commitments. But there is one more step you need to complete your Diabetes Mastery™.

Bridging the Diabetes Gap

Managing your diabetes is a lifelong responsibility, and your focus and diabetes management strategy will continue to evolve. Once you have successfully mastered one focus area in your Wheel of Diabetes Mastery™, you will need to repeat steps 2 to

6 to make progress in the next focus area, and so on. As you make progress, your horizon will move.

Your life's journey with diabetes is like a hike. When you start out walking, all you see at the end of the horizon is a hill. Once you have reached the top, your horizon expands, and you may see a beautiful valley with yet another hill or mountain to climb on the other side. The farther you get, the more your horizon extends.

There will always be another goal for you that is your hill or mountain to climb. We humans are bound to grow personally, professionally, and spiritually. Your immediate goal today may be to get your A1c down to 7.0. Once you have achieved that, your next target may be to get it down to 6.5. Or maybe you were happy with 7.0 for a while but now want to shift gears to advance your career. Getting your blood sugar in check is really just the catalyst for creating a beautiful life. Thank you, diabetes.

The space between where you are today and where you want to be is called the gap. Keep on bridging the gap and you will make changes in all focus areas of your life.

Staying Alive

I know from experience that despite our best-laid plans to reach our next destination, our bodies will become less forgiving as we grow older, and the sins from youth will creep up.

One day I began to feel pain in my groin that would not go away for weeks. Instead, it increased, and I suspected a urinary tract infection because the pain radiated up to my hips. My doctor first thought so, too, but it turned out to be advanced osteoarthritis. The fracture from my accident at age 3 left a spur that caused a hip impingement and damaged the cartilage. Decades of playing Frisbee and squash, practicing martial arts, and doing aggressive Rollerblading did not help matters. At 50, my hip needs to be replaced.

My goal is to push off surgery until I am in my 60s, because artificial hips only last about 20 years and also come with potential severe short- and long-term side effects. I intend to live well into my 90s, so the longer I can push off surgery, the better. Which is why I traded the boxing gloves for a yoga mat.

You, too, will eventually have issues, or you may already have them. As a person with diabetes, you are more prone to developing problems, such as heart disease, nerve and eye damage, and even Alzheimer's, than people without a chronic disease. Embracing a diabetic lifestyle can support you in preventing such complications.

Pumping Blood

As a person with diabetes, you are at an increased risk of heart disease and stroke, even with your blood sugar in check. You are two to four times more likely to die from heart disease than adults without diabetes. On average, 610,000 people die of heart disease in the United States every year; that's one in every four deaths. In addition, 80% of diabetics' deaths are due to heart disease, which can occur without any apparent symptoms. You may not feel it and, so you won't be able to report it in time. You may suddenly feel breathless, with your heart pumping faster or slower, and then die.

Your heart will need your absolute attention. As long as it pumps blood strongly enough, you'll live. Keep it pumping. Having a good cardiologist on your diabetes care team is not a luxury but a necessity. Consult with them regularly.

Movement is essential to your heart health. It ensures that your heart pumps blood full of oxygen to your lungs, blood vessels, and muscles. A healthy diabetic lifestyle includes walking, biking, swimming, yoga, or dancing. There is no need for excessive exercises, such as Spinning classes. Continuous moderate movement performed for at least 30 minutes 5 times a week is often enough. A brisk walk around the block for a half hour each day will reduce your risk of heart disease and obesity. No need to pump weights at the gym to keep your heart pumping blood.

If you can exercise at 70% of your heart rate, you won't feel exhausted. There are multiple ways of calculating your optimal heart rate, and it is typically much lower than we think. For me, it is around 138, which most people get to quickly with a brisk walk. There is no need to run on a treadmill. You can find your target heart rate on the website of the American Heart Association [5] or Google "optimal heart rate" for other resources.

If it is hard for you to find the extra time for a workout, then build movement into your daily routine with these simple strategies:

- Practice Egoscue anywhere. Exercise every morning after waking up and multiple times during the day. Find instructions on the resource page for this book: http://BloodSugarInCheck.com.

- Skip the elevator or escalator and walk up the stairs.

- Brush your teeth on one foot.

- Park your car as far away from the store as you can.

- Use technology and ask your smartphone to remind you to stand up and walk every 50 minutes.

- Get a standing desk; avoid sitting as much as you can.

- Stand up during conference calls.

- When you sit, lift your shoulders to your ears, tighten your core, and squeeze your butt.

---

[5] Target Heart Rates from the American Heart Association
https://www.heart.org/en/healthy-living/fitness/fitness-basics/target-heart-rates

- Get a dog. You will need to get them out of the house to poop and pee, rain or shine. Yes, it's annoying, but that's the idea.

- Put some music on and dance.

- Perform 5–10 squats in the bathroom stall, until the toilet finishes filling with water.

- Vacuum or sweep for an hour; it'll burn 150 calories.

- Instead of meeting friends for happy hour after work, play Frisbee in the park together.

- Instead of emailing your colleague across the cubicle farm, walk over and chat in person.

Vitalizing Your Cells

Your heart pumps blood to supply the cells in your body with oxygen and nutrients. Keeping it pumping is your first order of business; filling your blood with oxygen is the second.

Cells are living organisms that need three conditions to survive:

1. **Oxygen** Your cells use the oxygen you breathe to break down sugar. When glucose from your blood enters the cell, it uses oxygen to make energy. This process is called cellular respiration and drives many processes in your

cells, such as muscle contraction and how well your glands and nerves work.

High blood sugar weakens the walls of the small blood vessels and reduces the amount of oxygen and nutrients the cells receive. Because our blood sugar is always a bit high, even when it is well in check, we diabetics have an increased risk of nerve damage that can cause many serious complications, such as joint damage, urinary tract infections, sexual dysfunction, loss of a toe, foot, or leg, and more. We need to be especially aware of our cell health. Driving more oxygen into the cell is a must, not a should, for us.

2. **Water** Your cells need water for respiration. Without it, cells cannot move waste and by-products from energy production and take in nutrients. You need water for filtering and flushing out toxins. If you don't drink enough water, your cells won't work as well as they could. This is the reason dehydration shows first as loss of energy, not thirst. Just a 5% drop in bodily fluids can cause a 30% reduction in energy.

When you are dehydrated, cells cannot detox, and the many traces of chemicals in the cells delay and distort their ability to signal. Eventually, the nerves either lose their ability to transmit information, which shows as numbness, or start sending false signals, and you feel pain and tingling. After a while, this misfiring of the nerves can get so bad that people are unable to move. Some people get to a point where they would rather have a limb amputated than continue to live with the pain.

3. **Nutrients** All cells require amino acids from protein, essential fatty acids, glucose, minerals, vitamins, trace elements, and antioxidants. Magnesium, for example, helps you detoxify and keeps your immune system in top shape and your heart healthy. Antioxidants help cell repair, and potassium balances fluid levels, nerve function, and nutrient transport in the body. Vitamin B12 is essential for maintaining healthy nerve function. Placebo-controlled trials have shown that acetyl-L-carnitine, a naturally occurring amino acid, improves pain and nerve regeneration in patients with chronic diabetic neuropathy.

Drinking enough water is essential for your health. Most people can only go without water for only 3 days before they die, because the body starts to lose water from the blood first, and transportation of oxygen slows or even stops. A water loss of 9–12% triggers the organs in the body to begin a shut down.

Dehydration begins with unexplained tiredness; thirst comes second; and then you experience headaches, general discomfort, loss of appetite, confusion, purple fingernails, and seizures. Eventually, you will lapse into unconsciousness and die. People over 50 die more easily in hot weather because their sensation for thirst diminishes with age, and when hot weather hits, they are already dehydrated. The sun is just doing the rest.

When your blood sugar is high, your kidneys move excess sugar into your urine, dragging along fluids from your tissues. This triggers more frequent urination, which may leave you dehydrated also. Because your blood sugar is always on the high side, you are at an increased risk of being dehydrated.

Water is essential to life, and as a person with diabetes, you especially need to get lots of it. There are two ways you can hydrate:

- Drink: 70–80% of our water intake comes from drinking water and other beverages

- Eat: 20–30% of our water intake comes from food

How much you need to eat and drink depends on multiple factors, and I could fill an entire new book with that. For now, just note that drinking water and eating water-based foods are your two main ways of hydrating. Likewise, there are drinks and foods that dehydrate you and work against you, such as coffee, alcohol, sugar, salt, and cured meats.

As diabetics, we need to avoid:

- Alcohol
- Artichokes
- Asparagus
- Beets
- Bread
- Canned food
- Coconut water
- Coffee
- Cured meats
- Detox tea
- Energy drinks
- Fried foods
- Frozen dinners
- Fruit juice
- High-protein meals
- Pancakes
- Salty snacks
- Soda, including diet versions
- Soy sauce
- Waffle mixes

What's left for you to eat, you might ask? Read on.

Filling Up On Greens

Because the blood sugar of people with diabetes is always a bit higher than it should be, even when it is generally in check, we need to counterbalance the toxicity that it causes in our cells. The best way of doing that is by eating water-based vegetables and fruits that are low in sugar.

The jury is still out on if going fully vegan is a good thing. Growing research indicates eating meat regularly increases the risk of heart disease by up to 60%, while plant-based proteins are beneficial. On the other hand, you will need to take a supplement or look for foods fortified with vitamin B12 if you totally cut out animal products. This makes a case for the need for animal protein.

Then again, a clinical trial sponsored by NYU Langone Health attesting a vegan diet on heart patients found that a vegan diet was better at lowering one risk factor for heart attacks than the meal plan the American Heart Association recommends, which allows for modest amounts of sirloin steak, pork chops, chicken, fish, eggs, and low-fat dairy products.

While the link between red meat and heart disease is evident, the debate about dairy is more heated. Some studies say milk products are harmful; others state low-fat dairy is right for your heart; still others provide evidence that only whole fat milk protects the heart. Who should you believe? This is such an important issue, especially for us diabetics. Which basket shall we put our eggs into? Is it worth it to take a risk either way?

Some recent research suggests that the current advice from cardiologists to limit dairy intake should be reconsidered, because the evidence of a link to heart disease is inconsistent. For people with diabetes, the debate is doubly meaningful because of conflicting reports on the connection between cow milk and type 1 diabetes, as well as dairy products and their effect on people with type 2 diabetes.

When you start following the research, you can get confused easily. You will find strong evidence for and against all types of nutritional guidance. And because I like it simple, here are my rules for eating healthily.

Do

1. Eat as close to life as you can. Salad, vegetables, and fruits fall into that category. All kinds of meat, by definition, are dead. Processed meat is deader.

2. Soybeans/tofu, nuts, seeds, and legumes are all fair game.

3. Buy and eat local and organic.

Dump

1. All dairy food and beverages. Would you drink human breast milk? If your answer is no, then what makes you think that drinking the milk from a cow is a good idea?

2. Avoid all foods that dehydrate you.

3. Avoid all white foods, which spike your blood sugar: potatoes, rice, noodles, white bread, sugar.

Sometimes I believe that I have tried every diet in the world: low carb, high carb, high protein, keto, vegan, Atkins, fruit, juicing, HCG, *Nutrisystem*, *Body for Life*, *Eat This, Not That!*, blood type, Paleo, and intermittent fasting. They all worked. Even the HCG diet, which is highly controversial and especially not recommended for people with type 1 diabetes, worked very well for me. I lost 20 pounds in 1 month. The only diet that did not work for me was juicing. My wife, Ann, and I tried it once, and she loved it. I, who had not had problems with living on 500 calories per day for a month, did not make it through one day.

We are all different. You will need to make your own choices in collaboration with your diabetes care team. Almost all experts, however, agree on the benefits of eating water-based vegetables, green salad, and low-glycemic fruits as well as drinking water and moderately exercising on a regular basis. The adverse effects on your health from eating processed food, eating red meat, and sitting at your desk all day are also relatively clear. So, this is my starting point for a healthy diet. The rest is negotiable.

As for me, with a 50% blockage in one of my arteries, I am not taking any chances and have decided to go all vegan with an alkaline diet. I have a 7-year-old boy who needs me to be healthy for a long time, so no more messing around. But I also know that we can zigzag. We do not have to do it right all of the time. Remember to enjoy life. Let's celebrate ourselves. I found that an alkaline diet has a significant effect on my blood sugar management, but I also enjoy a scoop of ice cream or a piece of chocolate once in a while. Be kind to yourself too.

The alkaline diet is also controversial, because the body already does a good job of staying slightly alkaline. However, the purpose of following an alkaline diet is not to fight acidity but to make it easier for the body. In my mind, it is already hard enough for it to deal with high blood sugar.

An alkaline diet is also hard to follow. No meat, no dairy, no white stuff, no bread, no alcohol, no caffeine, and some other restrictions make it hard to implement, especially during travel. At the time of this writing, I have been traveling for business for 4 weeks, and in some places I have had to rely on junk food. As a result, I gained weight and developed a skin rash and cold sores. This never happens when I strictly follow an alkaline diet, but we often have no choice than to pivot. As soon as I am home, in about a week, I will be back to green smoothies in the morning, fresh food throughout the day, and shedding the pounds. Zigzag.

Savoring and Cherishing Fat

The nonfat diets have done us diabetics more harm than good. Nonfat often means double sugar or the presence of other harmful additives. For example, granola is very often labeled on the package as low in fat and fortified with vitamins and minerals. And its makers tout the "whole grains" in it. They forget to tell you that the average cereal brand includes about 25% white table sugar plus corn syrup, honey, fructose, and other ingredients that spike your blood sugar. The same is true for low-fat salad dressings, low-fat yogurt, reduced fat peanut butter—low-fat almost anything, really.

Have you ever wondered what replaces the fat in yogurt and cheese? Food manufacturers pour substitutes into their products to make it hold together and taste better, including sugar, flour, thickeners, unsaturated vegetable oils, carrageenan, sucrose polyesters, guar gum, esterified propoxylated glycerol, altered triglycerides, polydextrose, pectin, modified whey protein concentrate, microparticulate protein, and salt. Some of these fat substitutes cause problems. Your body will digest many of them only partially or sometimes not at all. Others have adverse effects on your digestive system or the bacteria in your colon.

The truth is that we all need fat in our diet, especially the kinds we find in nuts and seeds. They are important for maintaining healthy blood vessels and hormones. Omega-3s raise levels of a hormone called adiponectin, which increases insulin sensitivity. They also help reduce inflammation, prevent heart disease and stroke, and decrease insulin resistance.

Fat has gotten a bad reputation over the past few decades, mostly because of the negative impact on our health from saturated fats and trans fats. But not all fats are equal. Udo

Erasmus explained that very well in his book *Fats That Heal Fats That Kill*. In short, only omega-3fats and omega-6fats are considered essential, which means that if you do not get enough of them, you can become sick. Udo sees it this way: "A nonfat diet will eventually kill you, because you will not be getting those two essential nutrients from fats or from oils."

Omega-3 and omega-6 fats also play important roles in processes like blood clotting and inflammation. Here is where it becomes a bit confusing for us laymen. Omega-6s are pro-inflammatory, while omega-3s are anti-inflammatory. Neither is good or bad, per se. On the one hand, inflammation is good, as it protects our bodies from infection and, therefore, supports our survival. But it can also harm us. Chronic inflammation is linked to heart disease, metabolic syndrome, diabetes, arthritis, Alzheimer's, and many types of cancer.

So...what to do?

Erasmus has observed that balance matters. He believes that we have "too little omega-3 in our diets [and] far too much omega-6 in our bodies." His recommendation: "Get your omega-3s. They have to be in balance with the omega-6s. They should be both undamaged, made with health in mind. And you take a tablespoon per 50 pounds of body weight per day, and you mix it in food, spread it out over the course of the day, and you never use it for cooking. It's a replacement for the cooking oils, but you should've never cooked with the cooking oils either."

Adding the Good Stuff

Embracing a healthy lifestyle as a diabetic needs work. It does not come easily, especially away from home. There is almost nothing healthy to eat in fast food restaurants, for example. Apart from garden salads, everything else literally kills us. And I am not so sure about the salads there, either, given the many recent E. coli outbreaks in romaine lettuce and spinach. Even coffee shops are full of sugary, fatty cookies, brownies, cakes, and other sweets that we need to stay away from.

So much of what we eat on the go is either radiated, pasteurized, processed, preserved, or treated with pesticides. Whatsonmyfood.org found 54 different pesticides on spinach and 47 residues on apples. Many are taken in by the roots and distributed throughout the plants, so no amount of washing will remove them.

A number of these fruits and vegetables are cultivated to grow faster and yield more. As a result, they have about 30% less protein, calcium, potassium, iron, and vitamins B2 and C than they did in the year 1950. In addition, most produce loses 30% of its nutrients within 3 days of harvest. Vegetables can lose 15–55% of vitamin C within a week, and spinach can lose 90% within the first 24 hours. Steaming and boiling causes an additional 50% loss of vitamin C in broccoli, spinach, and lettuce. And for the carnivores amongst us, simmering and barbecuing meat destroys up to 60% of thiamin, niacin, and other B vitamins.

Going green alone is not enough. Ideally, we should buy our fresh fruits and vegetables not in the supermarket but from local organic farms right after they have been harvested. Although I highly recommend buying local, it is not practical for most of us, and it is also time-consuming, more labor intensive, and more expensive.

The long and short of it is that you will need to add essential nutrients to your diet to live healthily. Our food supply chain alone does not nourish us anymore. It helps us stay alive at best. Remember from Step 1 in this program that the human brain and body are programmed for survival. To thrive, you will need to wrestle your brain. Steps 2 to 6 help you do just that. Here in Step 7, you'll hack the food system and make sure your brain and body get the energy you need to stick with and succeed on your new plans.

We need supplements. We cannot do it without them. It is impossible, unless we get off the grid and farm organic food ourselves. But don't make a mistake and buy multivitamins at the supermarket or even from the local health food store. Study after study shows that there are no benefits from multivitamins in protecting the brain or heart. Controlled trials found that taking multivitamins, vitamin D, calcium, and vitamin C do not help in the prevention of cardiovascular disease, heart attack, stroke, or premature death. Vitamin E, once promoted as heart healthy, actually increases your risk of heart failure and prostate cancer.

There is no nice way of saying it, so I'll just do it bluntly: Multivitamins do not prevent cancer and heart disease. St John's wort will do nothing for your depression. Echinacea will not cure your common cold.

To make matters worse, there is little regulatory oversight in the supplement industry. Some even include contaminants that pose serious health risks to you, such as microbes, heavy metals, and toxins. Other supplements include more than 10 times the recommended intake of certain vitamins, which can be very risky to consume. High doses of vitamin E and A can increase the risk of cancer. Herbal and dietary supplements can cause liver toxicity.

But there is hope:

- Zinc has been linked to shortening the effects of a cold.

- Folic acid and B vitamins reduce the risk of cardiovascular disease and stroke.

- Controlled trials showed that adults who took vitamin D supplements daily lived longer than those who didn't.

- Probiotics improve glucose metabolism, especially when multiple species are taken and for longer than 8 weeks.

- Acetyl-L-carnitine improves pain, nerve regeneration, and vibratory perception in patients with chronic diabetic neuropathy.

- CoQ10 helps decrease heart disease by boosting energy production within heart muscle cells, preventing blood clots from forming, and acting as an antioxidant. There is also indication that it helps get your blood sugar in check.

- Alpha-lipoic acid supplements can improve insulin resistance and nerve damage caused by diabetes. They seem to reduce pain, tingling, and prickling in the feet and legs and may also help protect the retina from some of the damage caused by high blood sugar.

- Essential oils support the treatment of some complications of diabetes, such as gastrointestinal issues, weight gain, or diabetic neuropathy. They also help reduce diabetes-related stress.

You can find a list of all my recommended supplements here: http://www.bloodsugarincheck.com.

On the following pages you will find my favorite ones that have benefited me the most.

Vitamins et al

Vegan Lifelong Vitality Pack from DoTerra

This increases your health on the cellular level and includes almost all the vitamins, minerals, and supplements that have been proven to be effective in supporting your diabetes health, including acetyl-L-carnitine, alpha-lipoic acid, CoQ10, a complex of B vitamins, natural vitamin D, and zinc. It also includes a class of antioxidant molecules that protect against free-radical damage to cellular DNA, mitochondria, and other critical cell structures.

If you can only afford one dietary supplement, then this power pack is it.

Pure Synergy Super B-Complex

I take this B-vitamin complex in addition to the Vegan Lifelong Vitality Pack. Vitamin B is the most important supplement one can take as a vegan. This product is made with whole organic foods and is not isolated, synthesized, or corrupted with harmful chemicals. Pure Synergy is one of my all-time favorite brands, in large part because founder Mitchell May stands behind it.

Most multivitamins are nothing but synthetic ingredients, mostly made in China. Because your body cannot store water-soluble B vitamins, most supplements flush through your system in a couple of hours. Not this one. The Synergy Company uses only non-GMO, whole-food-based ingredients. This product is made with wholesome organic veggies and fruits that are then activated with enzymes and probiotics and slowly release into your system.

Udo's Choice Ultimate Oil Blend

Udo's oil is the perfect ratio of 2:1:1 of omega-3, -6, and -9 fatty acids. It is also completely vegan, which makes it compatible with an alkaline diet. The blend consists of nine organic ingredients, including flaxseed oil for the omega-3s, sunflower seeds to balance the omega-6s, evening primrose oil for the antioxidants, as well as coconut oil, rice/oat germ oil, GMO-free lecithin, and Vitamin E.

Pure Synergy USDA Organic Green Superfood

I cannot state it often enough. Eating greens is more important than eating fruits. Six studies involving more than 220,000 people concluded that eating one and a half servings of green leafy vegetables per day reduces the risk of type 2 diabetes by 14%. Eating more fruits and vegetables combined did not seem to have the same effect.

The exact reasons are not known. However, green leafy veggies may reduce the risk of getting type 2 diabetes because of their high concentrations of polyphenols and their antioxidant properties.

My research indicates that Pure Synergy offers the most comprehensive and trusted certified organic green superfood. It is also available in capsules for when you are on the go. Both include over 60 certified organic superfoods from aquatic greens, grass juices, sprouts to mushrooms and herbal extracts. Equally important: no fillers, fibers, additives, preservatives, sweeteners, or natural flavors.

Probiotics

I go back and forth with probiotics. Some of the highest-rated probiotics have not done anything for me, while others worked wonders. The most important thing to remember is that our bodies are all different. What works for me might not necessarily work for you. This appears to be especially true when it comes to probiotics. My advice is to find whatever works for your body and stick with it.

My practice is to change them every month, though I get conflicting information on whether it is necessary to rotate probiotic supplements. I do want you to make sure, though, that your probiotics are non-GMO, gluten free, yeast free, sugar free, wheat free, and nut free and do not include chemicals, preservatives, artificial colors, or artificial flavors. Here are two brands that are a good starting point:

DoTerra PB Assist+

This proprietary formula of prebiotic fiber and six strains of probiotic microorganisms delivers 6 billion CFUs (colony-forming units) of active probiotic cultures to your gut. It is also full of soluble prebiotic FOS (fructooligosaccharides) that feed the friendly bacteria. It has a double-capsule delivery system that makes sure the cultures are protected from stomach acid and get to where they are needed.

Udo's Choice Super 8 Hi-Potency Probiotic

While this blend does not have a double-capsule delivery mechanism, it includes live probiotic strains of the highest survivability and colonization rates. This means they can reach your intestines at full potency.

Heart and Eye Protector

Pure Synergy Eye Protector

My optometrist once detected an early sign of retinopathy in one of my eyes. That's when I did my research and discovered this product. Six months later, all signs of possible damage to my nerves disappeared. A few years later, there is still not the slightest indication of nerve damage to my eyes. Reviews online are just as glowing. Unfortunately, the Pure Synergy Eye Protector is either hard to get or only available at a premium outside of the United States. So, I stock up whenever I am home.

Pure Synergy Organic Heart Protector

Inspired by the Mediterranean and Okinawan diets, this supplement features heart-healthy nutrients. It may help with lowering your cholesterol and blood pressure. I have no scientific evidence that it works, but ever since I started taking it, I can feel my blood flowing and my heart pumping stronger.

Getting Oiled

You cannot cure your diabetes with essential oils, nor do they force your blood sugar up or down. But they can work wonders in relieving some common diabetes symptoms, especially for skin care and stress management. Essential oils can be inhaled, diffused, ingested, or even rubbed directly onto the skin, often on the bottom of the feet or back of the neck. Here are my favorites.

Frankincense Essential Oil

The king of oils, frankincense is known to support healthy cellular function and promote feelings of peace, relaxation, satisfaction, and overall wellness. It stimulates the immune system and may also help balance blood sugar, because high blood sugar often affects the immune system and vice versa.

Frankincense has a calming effect and antiseptic properties. Some people claim that frankincense helps scars fade more quickly, but I have never used it for that purpose. It does give me feelings of peace, relaxation, and satisfaction, which you may like after worrying about your blood sugar all day.

Lavender Essential Oil

Lavender is one the most popular essential oils, and I agree. It helps me sleep like a baby and has also been helpful in reducing my feelings of stress and increasing my concentration. It may also be a great choice when you first notice signs of diabetes burnout. Lavender essential oil has also been proven to help with chronic skin conditions, such as slow-healing ulcers.

Lemon Essential Oil

I use lemon oil throughout the day. Shortly after waking up, I take two drops in water and start alkalizing, flushing out toxins, and supporting my liver with simple and natural detoxification. It is also uplifting and encourages a happy spirit and good concentration.

Lemon oil also stimulates white blood cells, thus increasing our ability to fight off diseases, and improves blood circulation.

I ingest a few drops during the day. I am usually very cautious about swallowing essential oils, because some of them can be very potent, and even one drop can be too much for some. But this one is hard to overdose on, although of it may cause you to poop a lot.

DoTerra OnGuard Essential Oil Blend

On Guard is an excellent way to boost your immune system and shorten colds. My family uses it in winter in multiple ways, and we rarely get sick, even if the world around us has the sniffles. 'Nuff said.

Own Your Diabetes Mastery™

I have shared a number of tactics and practical tips with you that work for me and my clients, friends, and family. I believe these to be a good starting point for you as well. In the end, I want you to work with your diabetes care team and assemble your own way of eating that benefits your long-term diabetes health, develop your own day-to-day workout regimen, and find the combination of supplements that helps you feel your best.

Other pieces of advice are universally true. There are a few things I want you to remember and incorporate into your Diabetes Mastery™. In particular, drink enough water, eat water-based fruits and vegetables, and fill up on greens. Also make movement a priority. Your body is made to move.

CHAPTER ELEVEN

Practical Hacks for Blood Sugar Success

Preempt That Apology

Your friends and family love you no matter what. Over time, they will be able to tell when your blood sugar is low before you notice it yourself. They probably put up with more mood swings from you than you will ever know.

Acknowledge their patience and grace more often. You can do that in advance. Just tell them over dinner or a coffee klatch, "If I start acting out of character or become aggressive for no reason, it might be because my blood sugar level is very low or very high. Try not to take it personally. If you think my blood sugar is low, tell me. I will appreciate that. In either case, I apologize in advance if I act mean and nasty, and I truly appreciate your love and support."

(Thank you to Allice Keely Brownfield for the inspiration.)

I have asked family and friends to not just come by my house unannounced. Their timing may not be right because I am either dealing with low or high blood sugar; and I prefer to deal with it without the pressure of having to be sociable.

Get a Dog

Regular exercise is an important element of diabetes management. Your body is made for movement, not sitting. Getting a dog is a surefire way to get out of the house every day, rain or shine. They also make you feel good by welcoming you like a long-lost friend each time you enter the house. Cats do not give you any of those benefits. Get a dog.

Take the Lemon

Skip the soda. When eating out, order water and ask for lemon wedges on the side. Every half decent restaurant has lemons. Squeeze the juice into the water. Voila, you have your alkalizing drink. You will also avoid ingesting the nasty stuff in diet soda, such as caffeine, glutamate, aspartate, phosphoric acid, and chemicals found in rust remover, steel cleaner, and cement. Drink water with lemon instead.

Use Siri or Alexa

Your day can quickly get busy, and you can easily become distracted and forget to check your blood sugar, take your medication, or even get off the chair to breathe. Use technology to remind you of these tasks. Tell Alexa, "Remind me to inject my insulin at 10 p.m." or ask Siri to remind you to measure your blood sugar every 2 hours. Of course, any smart device will do.

Kolbe Each Other

Have your significant other take the Kolbe A™ Index test and then get a Takes Two℠ report or Comparisons: A to A™ report. Kolbe Takes Two℠ is a fun, fast, and easy way to bring more joy and less stress to your relationship. You will get personalized tips to help you get along better, learn what to let go of, and learn what to hold onto. The Kolbe Comparison: A to A™ report tells you how you work together if there is conative stress between you and how to avoid it. That's why I make the big decisions in my household and my wife, Ann, makes the small decisions. Which decisions are big or small, Ann decides.

Bring Your Beans

Always have jelly beans with you. Put them into smaller bags and have them everywhere: your car, jacket, gym bag, office, etc.

When your blood sugar drops, you'll want to have these little lifesavers ready. Be careful not to eat too many, which will spike your blood sugar. Keep them in small containers in 15-carb amounts. Do not use Skittles, as they tend to be harder to chew and swallow. Jelly beans are easier to gobble down. You can also use chewable glucose tablets, but they may end up being more expensive than jelly beans. A tube of 10 glucose tablets can cost from $1.50 to $6.50. That is between $20 and $81 for a pound of sugar. Other options are glucose gels and chews. But they are equally expensive, and some come with warnings like: "Consuming this product can expose you to chemicals including lead, which are known to the State of California to cause cancer."

Overcome the Needle

Many people have a genuine fear of needles. That's not the best fear to have when you have diabetes, which requires you to use them every day, either to prick your finger or inject insulin. Advanced clinical hypnotherapy and neuro-linguistic programming (NLP) can help you overcome your fear, sometimes after only two sessions.

Fly with Essentials

Going international or flying across multiple time zones is not easy for anyone—even for healthy people who fly first class. Having diabetes and an economy seat in the back of the plane makes matters worse. Service begins an hour or so after takeoff. Before cabin crews roll out their carts to get you a drink, your tongue is most likely already glued to the roof of your mouth. Bring plenty of water on board. Yes, it costs a fortune at airports, but your kidneys, liver, and heart will thank you. Also, bring food that you like. Unless you fly business, there is never enough food on your tray to get you across the Atlantic. And those hot, greasy ham and cheese sandwiches they give you before landing? There is only one place to put them: in the trash bin. Order a special vegan meal ahead of time for international flights and you will often get fresh fruit instead.

Beat the Jet Lag

This one is hard. Flying across time zones takes a toll on everyone. Once you arrive at your destination, the time of day no longer lines up with your body's internal clock. It can take 3 days or longer before you feel like yourself again. For people with diabetes, traveling across multiple time zones can increase the risk of hypoglycemia. You will need to consult with your diabetes care team about what to do. The advice you receive will differ for westbound travel (days are longer) and eastbound travel (days are shorter). An excellent resource to start at is http://diabetestravel.org/time-zones.

Take Some Air

Deep breathing for 3 minutes, followed by pushups and then a cold shower, does wonders for stabilizing your diabetes. But beware of nutcases who tell you that breathing cures diabetes. It cannot. But proper breathing does help alleviate symptoms of a host of illnesses, such as multiple sclerosis, arthritis, diabetes, clinical depression, anxiety, bipolar disorder, and cancer. Dutch extreme athlete Wim Hof took it a few steps further and proved scientifically that breathing can influence even your autonomous nervous system. A study published in the *Proceedings of the National Academy of Sciences of the United States of America* states that by consciously hyperventilating, Hof can increase his heart rate, adrenaline levels, and blood alkalinity. Maybe it's not so nuts after all. https://www.wimhofmethod.com.

Always Have Needles Handy

I cannot tell you how often I leave the house with my insulin pen but forget to bring needles. One time, I only brought a single needle with me, but it fell on the floor when I tried to screw it on, rendering it useless. I spent the entire evening at the restaurant on green leaves and water. It's healthy but not always what you want. I have learned to keep needles in my office, jackets, computer bag, and car. This is not the best practice, but during times when I urgently need a needle, I am always very grateful for all the extras that I can find.

Keep Your Insulin Cool

Keeping insulin chill in the heat can be a challenge if you don't have an ice pack or fridge nearby. Some people with diabetes use a Frio wallet to keep their insulin safe at hot temperatures. As for me, I have traveled to places such as Cameroon, Mozambique, Jamaica, Egypt, Greece, and Sicily without any gadgets, and my insulin has never gone bad or failed me. I usually just keep my pen in my front pocket and my stored insulin out of the sun. I figure that most insulin is relatively stable in warm weather and can be kept at room temperature for 28 days. It loses potency only at unusually high temperatures. Other than that, I don't spend much time or effort worrying about heat and insulin. I do make it a point, though, to store my insulin in the fridge whenever I can.

Check with the maker of your insulin to find out their temperature guidelines. If you have a pump, then you will need to check with its manufacturer as well.

Want to see an updated list of diabetes hacks or have one you want to share? Head over to my Facebook group.

CHAPTER TWELVE

Obstacles to Diabetes Mastery

By now, you have probably realized that keeping your blood sugar in check is a process. No single technique is the solution to your challenges. It is a way of life.

The Wheel of Diabetes Mastery™ gave you all the variables for your strategy to keep your blood sugar in check. Now it is all about continuous implementation. Easy, right? Until life gets in the way. A few things are likely to blindside you:

- You get "back to normal." The old forces inside you will keep on pulling you back into old habits for quite a while. You'll need regular returning for a few weeks to ensure you stay on track.

- You are out of flow. Many people confuse their conative strengths with what they like and as a result come to incorrect conclusions during the Flow Factor™ exercise. You will need to take a Kolbe A™ Index assessment and get a full interpretation of your report.

- Your triggers change. It is very common for another trigger to inconspicuously slip in once you've eliminated one trigger. For example, your trigger for eating chocolate may have been boredom at one time. Eventually, you feel like you deserve a treat each time you accomplish something significant, and soon enough a minor achievement—like coming home from work—is a trigger for celebration and indulging. You will need to be proactive in detecting and eliminating these triggers.

- You get frustrated. You will have times when nothing works. No matter what you do and how hard you try, your blood sugar won't come down or will keep on bouncing. You will need encouragement and individualized insights and guidance to pull through.

- You learn of long-term complications. Yes, it happens. Diabetes Mastery™ cannot undo the damage that has already been done. You will need additional support to make the best of your situation. Remember Nick Vujicic, who was born with no arms and no legs and now lives to inspire millions around the world with his story? Well, he also tried to kill himself at age 8 by drowning himself in a bathtub. What stopped him from going through with it was his love for his parents, and one day Nick's mother coached him with a story of a severely disabled man. That man's story made a significant impact on Nick. You will need help changing your story as well.

- A loved one needs your help, and you put yourself second. That happens to all of us, but it is not the best practice. There is a reason they tell you on airplanes that you must put on your own oxygen mask first when the cabin loses pressure. You cannot help the person next to you when you have passed out. You will need a reminder that you cannot be of help to someone unless you are strong first.

- You might lose your job and health insurance. We know that recessions come in cycles. No one really knows when the next one will come, but we all agree that it will. That's just how financial markets work. You will need to develop alternative strategies for managing your health.

- Your weight has increased. That usually happens over the holidays, on vacation, or during periods of unusual stress. Or sometimes for no apparent reason. But it makes you wonder why you went through all the effort in the first place, and you may want to give up altogether. You will need help getting back on track.

None of these obstacles are unique to you. We all face them, and the good news is that there are proven strategies to overcome them. You cannot let your happiness and well-being be dependent on elements that you cannot control. There is always going to be something, or someone, that stands in the way of your joy, whether it is the person who sits in the White House, the weather, the economy, or diabetes. What they all have in common is that you cannot control them. You can only exercise influence, and sometimes even that option is not available. What you can control when life throws you curveballs is your focus. What are the things and people that you can influence? How can you make the best out of your situation when life sucks?

You can almost always control your thoughts, your focus, and your environment. I have learned from observation and experience that we become the people whom we surround ourselves with. In writing this book, I also have realized that very few people in my life have diabetes. The reason is that I have always seen myself as an athlete and achiever. I have never once seen myself as a diabetic first—or second or third. For me, diabetes has always been a minor inconvenience at worst.

My friends are business owners, executives, coaches, motivational speakers, yoga teachers, and martial artists. They are loving, caring, and engaged parents, daughters, sons, siblings, friends, and mentors. I would be totally happy if that were all that people said about me at my eulogy. But my point is that you, too, become whom you surround yourself with.

People with diabetes who have their blood sugar in check typically surrounded themselves with supportive, like-minded peers. They have a network of doctors who care for them and lift them up. They seek out friends who embrace healthy lifestyles and are nonjudgmental about their illness.

It is easy to find downhearted people, because being

miserable together makes life less painful. You will find sympathy and compassion from the people who feel your pain. But being with them does not lead to health, happiness, and sanity. It just makes your depression less lonely.

I am not suggesting that you abandon your friends and family. Love them, but find the additional support to help you on your way. To do that, you need:

- A support network

- A mentor who has already achieved more than you want

- A coach who can give you new insights, practical new skills, awareness, and knowledge

The most successful people get help from a coach. Scott Johnson, a type 1 diabetes blogger, was awarded the *Insulindependence 2013 Athletic Achievement Award* as a 'regular' person with diabetes who is working hard to take care of his health. He attributes his success to the help he received from Marcey Robinson, who coaches athletes with diabetes across the globe. "Oftentimes doctors and people with diabetes think it should be easy and straight-forward and get frustrated when it's not," Robinson says. "Just like diabetes management is individualized from person to person, the blood sugar–management strategy changes from exercise session to exercise session. There are multiple variables at play, and knowing that they exist and how to adjust for them is half the battle."

That's why I am offering the Diabetes Mastery™ coaching program, which speeds you on your path to greater health, happiness, and sanity with diabetes. This is by far the most life-changing thing I have ever created in my life and the fastest route to your success.

My wish for you is that you get your blood sugar in check so you can live the life you want and deserve. Blood sugar will always be on your mind, whether you are in a great mental state or a bad one, so you might as well make it a good one. Remember that when things do not go your way, you can alter your state by radically changing either your physiology or your focus.

This is often easier said than done. I successfully teach and coach hundreds of people and teams each year, but I still cannot fix myself. Just as a chiropractor needs another bone fixer to adjust their spine, a coach needs a coach. And so do you. Yes, you can make progress alone, but you can really excel only with the help of a coach and mentor.

Bill Gates, for example, needed Warren Buffett, and Mark Zuckerberg needed Steve Jobs. Virgin founder Richard Branson admits that he "wouldn't have [gotten] anywhere in the airline industry without the mentorship of Sir Freddie Laker, [and] going it alone is an admirable, but foolhardy and highly flawed approach to taking on the world."

Diabetes Mastery™ is an essential part of creating the life of your dreams. You also know by now that it is a two-way street.

You cannot be successful in your job, for example, without managing your blood sugar well, and it will be hard to stabilize your blood sugar if your job does not allow it.

This program has taken you far beyond pricking your fingers, counting your carbs, dosing your medication, and exercising. It has moved you from looking at diabetes as a technical problem to tackling the disease with your mind also. It has expanded your horizons and opened new possibilities, avenues, and ways of thinking about all aspects of your life.

Imagine what you could achieve, how far you could see, and how high you could reach if you had that kind of support and motivation in a one-on-one setting with an experienced mentor and coach. Do you see yourself pushing further than you ever thought you could?

If the answer is *yes*, then my 12-week Diabetes Mastery™ coaching program is your next step. Here are the first goals that my clients achieve during my program:

- **Create your plan to better health and happiness with diabetes.** I will help you align your need to avoid pain with your desire to gain pleasure, which we discussed in Step 1. You will prioritize your life by identifying your basic human needs and the support network that you will need to help you meet them.

- **Understand your life with diabetes with perspective to key relationships, joy, pains, and hopes.** We will create and discuss the Wheel of Diabetes Mastery™ you have created in Step 2 in more depth and detail. There is also a Wheel of Career Development™ and other tools that can help you get clarity and focus.

- **Live stress free and anxiety free with diabetes by staying energized and in flow.** Diabetes Mastery™ coaching includes interpretation of your natural talents and strengths so you can make deliberate decisions on the 20% of action that gives you 80% of the results. We discussed this approach in Step 3.

- **Gain in-depth insights into your natural talents and strengths and learn how to use them in your Diabetes Mastery™.** You will especially benefit from coaching when it comes to doctoring tasks with the guided version of the Flow Factor™ exercise from Step 4. These are the hardest to crack and often need an unbiased view.

- **Reverse engineer your goals and condition yourself for success.** You will begin to change your focus and beliefs, improve your physiology, and change the language in your head that holds you back. The neuro-associative conditioning from Step 5 happens here with additional exercises that make it last.

- **Find and eliminate unconstructive triggers and patterns that hold you back.** You will take a critical look at your crazy eights from Step 6, and together we will identify the triggers and unhealthy responses and replace them with healthy ones.

- **You and I will work on building healthy life choices into your daily routine.** We'll follow along the lines we touched on in Step 7, but in coaching sessions, we will find solutions for your unique situation. This is the most exciting part of the 12-week Diabetes Mastery™ coaching program. Here is where we'll make it fun and rewarding and find new possibilities, personal and professional growth, deeper relationships, and a higher meaning of life.

What would it mean to you if you knew you could achieve anything you wanted if you only put your mind to it? How would you live with diabetes if you knew you had your blood sugar in check? Which dreams could you live, relationships would you build and foster, spiritual awareness would you reach? How would your career blossom if you had the emotional strength, resilience, and confidence?

To inquire about diabetes mentorship, apply on my website at http://www.bloodsugarincheck.com.

Here is what people are saying about the effectiveness of my coaching programs and workshops:

- "Andrew is the mentor that gives the hero the supplies, knowledge, and confidence required to overcome his or her fear and face life's big adventure." —Anna K.

- "Andrew is a very experienced coach who knows his methods very well. With his help I could identify not only the areas where I will need more help in the future in order to be more effective, but also the ones I like the most." —Orsolya F.

- "I came out inspired, uplifted, and much more aware of who I am." —Isabelle D.

- "Andrew has an amazing ability to create an open atmosphere. He also pushed me to reflect on my situation and find my own answers, and I left with a clear and actionable plan." —Grainne O.

- "Andrew showed me how strong and confident I actually am. I thank him for showing me that I am a wonderful, strong, confident, beautiful person and a force to be reckoned with." —Anne F.

- "Life has been amazing, with no worrying and actually doing what has become a pure amazing life! I want to encourage everyone who requires help or guidance in their life to work with Andrew." —Mike C.

- "Andrew helped me to give myself permission to follow my passions, start something new, and write the first chapter of a new adventure— after just a few coaching sessions. I call that impactful leadership!" —Alaina B.

- "Andrew gave me great insight into how I will keep moving forward without doing the two-legged/feet driving. Brake then gas, break and gas!" —Eileen C.

Will you write the next success story? Apply for diabetes coaching here http://www.bloodsugarincheck.com.

This is the fastest way of achieving the results that you want. Period. How long can you afford to let your diabetes roller coaster go on? What will it cost you if you do not take action now?

Questions? Email me at andrew@bloodsugarincheck.com

Thank you for staying with me throughout the book. You have given me your most treasured gift: your time.

Work hard, be nice, and stay amazing.

Andrew Lawless

ACKNOWLEDGEMENTS

Thank you, Ann, my wife, my muse, my rock, keeper of all that is righteous in the Lawless family. Steady like a train, sharp like a knife. Without your support, I would not have been able to acquire the core skills, tools, techniques, and experience that made this book. You encouraged me to invest time and money at a moment when we could least afford it. Your unconditional love and unwavering belief in what I do have been the rock from which I continue to rise. Thank you for teaching me how to love.

Thank you, Dylan, for being the *bestest* younger son ever. For weeks, you have been so patient while I sat in front of my computer from morning to midnight to finish this book and take care of business. You are the most fabulous little big man I know. I especially loved your corn and spinach soup, which gave me more energy and inspiration. May you always keep your positive outlook on life and continue to make the best out of every situation. Stay amazing.

Thank you, Arian, my most favorite older son. You have been a great travel companion through life. I will always remember when you managed my doctors at the hospital in the Dominican Republic— all with one year of Spanish in school and at age 11. Very impressive. As you continue to grow strong in your life college, your success and health give hope to so many people and parents with type 1 diabetes. You are living proof that people with diabetes can raise extraordinary sons and daughters. Your very presence assures parents with this disease that their children will have fantastic, meaningful lives if they put their mind to it. Keep inspiring.

Thank you, Roxanne, for being my oldest and most steady travel companion, even—and especially as—my ex-wife. You are probably the one person who faced my mood swings from blood sugar roller coasters the most. Thank you for teaching me how to stay true to values and for your forgiveness and grace.

Thank you, Anne von Chamier, for being the first woman to show me that I can be loved, that I do have self-worth, and that I am marvelous, amazing, incredible, a dream come true like everyone else. We even rented Fortuna Duesseldorf's football stadium for the German Ultimate Frisbee Championship in 1985. That was a feat! You gave me the support I needed to develop the confidence that I now have to inspire onstage and in workshops.

Thank you, Dr. Douglas Frankel, for being the best physician any diabetic can dream of. Your proactive care and deep compassion have been a cornerstone of my diabetes health. You gave my wife, Ann, so much comfort, and she still appreciates your calling back on a Saturday night to check in. Everyone should have a doctor like you. I am deeply honored by your introducing me to your network of specialists.

Thank you, Dr. Lauren Rubin, for checking my eyes so thoroughly. I always thought that when my eyes are OK, so are my kidneys. Your care is world class. Because of that, I always wanted to give you a hug for everything you have done. So, here we go. Big German bear hugs from me.

Thank you, Dr. Michael Urban, for restoring my gum health and holding me accountable for keeping it up. I never knew that having professional deep cleanings can lower your HbA1c. I wish we would have met earlier.

Thank you, Dr. Eamonn Twoomey, fellow type 1 diabetic with an upbeat approach to care. When I moved to Ireland, my biggest worry was building a new diabetes care team. I am so grateful that someone of your magnitude practices in Lackagh. You are a hidden gem.

Thank you, Hanni Shereen Baya, for your inspiration in Egypt when the local diabetes association abandoned us and we were left without water in the desert. I will always remember you singing Chris de Burgh songs. Thank you for teaching me resilience.

Thank you, Udo Staggemeyer, Kerstin (Jentsch) Musweiler, and Jürgen Kowalek. You were like older siblings to me. I will always, always know that without your support I would not have become an athlete, martial artist, or musician. You looked out for me when I was young and no one else cared that much. Life is scary when you are a teenager with type 1 diabetes. You made it a little less cold and quite a hell of a bit warmer. Jürgen, thank you for letting me drive your Ford Taunus and program your Amstrad computer. You set the stage for my best-selling computer book. Also, thank you for letting me sleep on your couch when I got thrown out of the house in the middle of the night.

Thank you, Tony Robbins, for the many inspirational videos and books. Many of your teachings and insights appear in this book and my program in so many ways. You taught me that there is always a better way, and I am so grateful for being able to extend that message to my own readers.

Thank you, Magali and Mark Peysha, for introducing me to and certifying me in strategic intervention. The concepts that you taught me are changing my clients' lives every day. Fortunately/Unfortunately is a lifestyle and a choice. I am so privileged that you gave me the options, concepts, and strategies to take positive action.

Thank you, Kathy Kolbe, for certifying me as a consultant to spread your wisdom. The idea of having the freedom to be yourself is a key promise to myself. Your work will continue to make a difference in people with diabetes worldwide.

Thank you, Bruce Springsteen, for "Thunder Road."

ABOUT THE AUTHOR

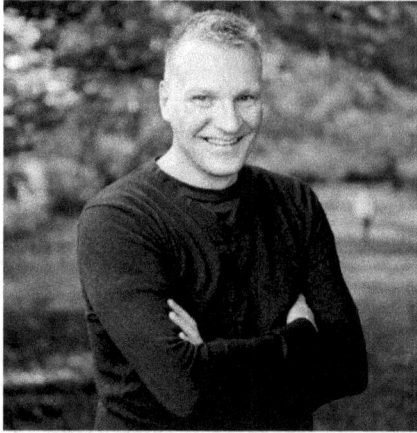

Andrew is a diabetes life coach. He has had type 1 diabetes for more than 40 years, with no signs of complications, and his mission is to enable other people with diabetes to keep their blood sugar in check so they won't lose a toe or kidney or die early. In short, Andrew wants you to be healthy and happy with your illness.

At the core of his work is strategic intervention, a coaching methodology developed by Tony Robbins and five partners. Andrew is certified by two of the codevelopers of this coaching framework, Magali and Mark Peysha. He is also certified in Kolbe Wisdom™ and is a finalist for the Kolbe Professional Award, which is given to top-tier coaches who have made a positive impact on people around the world by harnessing the power of their instinctive strengths.

Because of his own history and success with diabetes, Andrew is especially passionate about helping people with diabetes reach their dreams with their blood sugar in check. He has acquired the most successful tools and instruments from three decades of research and living with his illness.

Despite developing type 1 diabetes at age 11, his accomplishments include being one of Germany's top ten Frisbee players at age 19 in all disciplines; writing a national computer book best seller in Germany at age 23; emigrating to the United States at age 30 and eventually becoming a citizen; consulting with the FBI in defensive tactics; being headhunted by the World Bank in Washington, D.C.; and traveling to over 50 countries and working in 7 of them.

Professionally, Andrew has a unique blend of experience in behavioral sciences, publishing, digital marketing, and localization. His accomplishments range from managing a corporate turnaround of Berlitz in Central and Eastern Europe to transforming the World Bank's global approach to localizing its analytical work.

Andrew presented his successes to the Obama White House administration and testified before the US Senate on the importance of professional development. He served as a trainer and consultant to the FBI's Behavioral Science Unit, where he helped analyze the mindset of hostage takers. He served as an adjunct professor at the University of Maryland.

Andrew is also known for having followed Bruce Springsteen throughout Ireland. One challenge he is proud of mastering: keeping his blood sugar in check for 4 hours in front of the stage at a Springsteen concert in Limerick. One of Andrew's life goals is to meet The Boss in person to thank him for the song "Thunder Road." Without it, Andrew would not have made it out of his rundown neighborhood next to a glass factory and railway station.

Connect with Andrew on LinkedIn[6] or follow him on Facebook[7] and Twitter.[8]

Andrew can be contacted via email[9] or just visit his website.[10]

---

[6] LinkedIn *https://www.linkedin.com/in/lawlessandrew*
[7] Facebook *https://www.facebook.com/lawlessing*
[8] Twitter *https://twitter.com/bloodsugarcoach*
[9] Email: *andrew@bloodsugarincheck.com*
[10] Website: *https://teamlawless.com*

Keep On Living Large With Diabetes

Thank you for reading.

I am excited about your new steps to a happier and healthier life with diabetes. Getting your diabetes under control is a lifelong journey. I want to make sure you stay on course.

I know from my coaching clients that forces will want to pull you back, away from your new path. While this is normal, think about how your newly found love of diabetes has changed you. What would it mean to you and your loved ones if you lost that?

That's why I am offering you a tool kit of resources, including:

- Free and unlimited downloads of all diabetes success tools used in this book

- Access to the online companion course for greater health, happiness, and sanity with diabetes

- Access to my closed Facebook Diabetes Mentor group so you can connect with like-minded people with diabetes who lift you up

To get the free tool kit, join my Diabetes Mentor Facebook Group at *https://www.facebook.com/groups/diabetesmentor*

Work hard, be nice, and stay amazing.

Andrew Lawless | andrew@bloodsugarincheck.com